MALNUTRITION, ENVIRONMENT, and BEHAVIOR

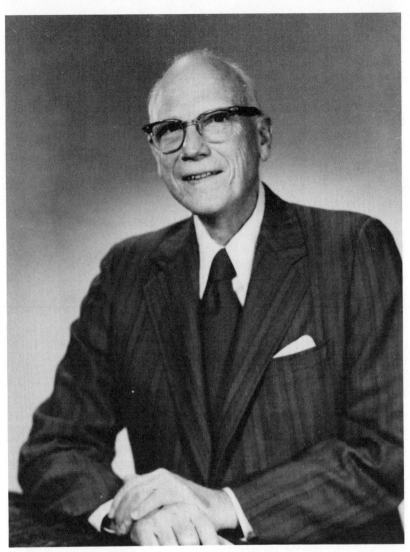

Richard H. Barnes

MALNUTRITION, ENVIRONMENT, and BEHAVIOR

New Perspectives

Edited by DAVID A. LEVITSKY

Cornell University Press ITHACA and LONDON

First published 1979 by Cornell University Press.
Published in the United Kingdom by Cornell University Press Ltd.,
2-4 Brook Street, London W1Y 1AA.

International Standard Book Number 0-8014-1045-2
Library of Congress Catalog Card Number 78-58016

Printed in the United States of America

*Librarians: Library of Congress cataloging information
appears on the last page of the book.*

*To Richard H. Barnes, scientist,
professor, dean*

An eternal source of inspiration

CONTENTS

Contents

PREFACE

This book reviews the changing hypotheses and concepts concerning the effect of malnutrition on mental development and provides a strongly critical discussion of current issues in the area of nutrition and behavior. The presentation of the essays in this book was organized with three major objectives in mind. First and foremost was the recognition of Richard H. Barnes, to whom this volume is dedicated, a man whose influence has profoundly affected both the research and the academic lives of so many of us in nutrition and the health sciences. He brought together in the laboratory and around the conference table researchers from many disciplines to talk and work on common problems. It seemed fitting on the eve of his retirement that we should assemble his colleagues and friends from many parts of the world and diverse areas of study to honor him.

A second objective was publicly to review experimental research and to assess progress over the past eight to ten years. In 1967, Nevin Scrimshaw organized a conference on Malnutrition, Learning, and Behavior at the Massachusetts Institute of Technology. This, one of the first international meetings on the subject, brought together researchers from all over the world to examine the relationship between malnutrition and mental development. At that time some research data seemed to indicate that malnutrition early in life caused mental retardation by structurally and irreversibly damaging the brain. This view was immediately picked up by both the scientific and the lay press. It should be noted, however, that several critics at the meeting challenged that conclusion. As we reexamine the problem after eight years of research on both animals and humans, we can see two shifts in approach. The most obvious change is that researchers are no longer talking about mental retardation; rather they emphasize behavioral changes induced by malnutrition. Second, they emphasize the role of the environment in the cognitive development of the mammal and, more important, the way malnutrition interferes with the interaction of the child with its environment.

A third objective was to discuss our data and open them to good scientific criticism. Interactions among scientists of different points of view will, we hope, provide new insights, stimulate ideas, and generate higher quality research. It is particularly important in multidisciplinary research that methods, data, and conclusions be tested by criticism from the many disciplines involved.

This book originated in the Proceedings of the Cornell Conference on Malnutrition and Behavior, held in November 1975. The chapters were prepared from manuscripts presented to the organizers prior to the conference and were revised for presentation here; the discussion material was prepared from tape recordings of the conference sessions. All of the material was edited for clarity and to eliminate repetition; however, some of the discussion material that was not germane to the subject of this book has not been included.

Organizing a conference and publishing its proceedings require help from many people. In particular, I thank Malden Nesheim, Director of the Division of Nutritional Sciences, Cornell University, for his assistance and encouragement. I am grateful to the College of Human Ecology (Cornell University), the National Institute of Child Health and Human Development (NICHD), Quaker Oats Company, The National Dairy Council, Ross Laboratories, and Mead Johnson Research Center for providing financial support for the conference and the preparation of the material. Finally, I express my personal thanks and appreciation to Margaret Dallyn for her help in arranging and executing the conference and editing the manuscript; to Doreen Doty for her assistance in preparing the manuscripts; and to Barbara Strupp for her time and effort in the final compilation of the manuscript.

DAVID A. LEVITSKY

Ithaca, New York

CONTRIBUTORS AND PARTICIPANTS

Richard H. Barnes, Cornell University, Ithaca, New York

David A. Blizard, New York University Medical Center, New York, New York

Charles Boelkins, Harvard School of Public Health, Boston, Massachusetts

Joseph Bronzino, Worcester Foundation for Experimental Biology, Shrewsbury, Massachusetts

Josef Brozek, Lehigh University, Bethlehem, Pennsylvania

Adolfo Chávez, National Institute of Nutrition, Mexico

David Coursin, St. Joseph Hospital, Lancaster, Pennsylvania

Joaquin Cravioto, Instituto Nacional de Ciencias y Tecnología, DIE, Mexico City; Andrew D. White Professor-at-Large, Cornell University, Ithaca, New York

Victor Denenberg, University of Connecticut, Storrs, Connecticut

John Dobbing, University of Manchester, Manchester, England

Herman Epstein, Brandeis University, Waltham, Massachusetts

John Fernstrom, Massachusetts Institute of Technology, Cambridge, Massachusetts

William B. Forbes, Worcester Foundation for Experimental Biology, Shrewsbury, Massachusetts

Slávka Fraňková, Institute for Clinical and Experimental Medicine, Prague, Czechoslovakia

Janina Galler, Boston University Medical Center, Boston, Massachusetts

E. J. Hawrylewicz, Mercy Hospital and Medical Center, Chicago, Illinois

Harry Jacobs, U.S. Army Natick Laboratory, Natick, Massachusetts

J. Kissane, Mercy Hospital and Medical Center, Chicago, Illinois

Robert Klein, INCAP, Guatemala

J. P. Leahy, Worcester Foundation for Experimental Biology, Shrewsbury, Massachusetts

Seymour Levine, Stanford University, Stanford, California

11

Contributors and Participants

David A. Levitsky, Cornell University, Ithaca, New York
Loy Lytle, Massachusetts Institute of Technology, Cambridge, Massachusetts
Celia Martínez, National Institute of Nutrition, Mexico
Thomas Massaro, Cornell University, Ithaca, New York
M. Miller, Worcester Foundation for Experimental Biology, Shrewsbury, Massachusetts
Peter Morgane, Worcester Foundation for Experimental Biology, Shrewsbury, Massachusetts
Martha Neuringer, Oregon Regional Primate Research Center, Beaverton, Oregon
Ernesto Pollitt, The University of Texas, Houston, Texas
Clark T. Randt, New York University Medical Center, New York, New York
Merrill S. Read, National Institute of Child Health and Human Development, Bethesda, Maryland
Oscar Resnick, Worcester Foundation for Experimental Biology, Shrewsbury, Massachusetts
Henry Ricciuti, Cornell University, Ithaca, New York
Stephen Richardson, Albert Einstein College of Medicine, Bronx, New York
Arthur J. Riopelle, Louisiana State University, Baton Rouge, Louisiana
David Rush, Columbia University, New York, New York
Kenneth Samonds, Harvard School of Public Health, Boston, Massachusetts
Maria Simonson, Johns Hopkins University School of Hygiene and Public Health, Baltimore, Maryland
James Smart, University of Manchester, Manchester, England
Warren Stern, Burroughs-Wellcome, Research Triangle Park, North Carolina
David Strobel, University of Montana, Missoula, Montana
Edith van Marthens, University of California, Los Angeles, California
Sandra Wiener, Stanford University School of Medicine, Stanford, California
Myron Winick, Columbia University, New York, New York
Stephen Zamenhof, University of California, Los Angeles, California

PART I

BACKGROUND

David Coursin **1**

Introduction

A major reason for holding the Cornell Conference on Malnutrition and Behavior was to assess the status of research, particularly that on animals, and its relevance to humans. By bringing together information from various investigators, we hoped to be able to identify where there is agreement and where there is disagreement. Beyond that, we hoped to determine the gaps in our knowledge so that we could move more fortuitously to fill them. Furthermore, it was important for us to determine the value of current methodologies and how to improve on their specificity and sensitivity as well as their standardization. Finally, we hoped to identify appropriate avenues for future research.

With all of these responsibilities in mind, it was most appropriate that the meeting to accomplish these tasks be held at Cornell University, primarily because of the presence at Cornell of Richard H. Barnes, a man who has been one of the pioneers and leaders in research in the field of nutrition, brain development, and behavior. Barnes has contributed immensely to the field not only through his personal research, but also by stimulating undergraduate and graduate student activities. He is responsible as well for having enlisted the talents of expert faculty members such as Henry Ricciuti and David Levitsky. Barnes's influence has spread across the world, and the guidelines and concepts that he has fostered are being well received everywhere; his interests and concepts have been major factors in research in both animals and humans.

One way to illustrate the importance of the conference is to provide a brief historical perspective from my own experiences. This is, first of all, a very young field with a significant history of less than twenty-five years standing. Except for a few giants of the past such as Benjamin Platt from the British Medical Research Council; R. F. A. Dean from Africa; Herbert Birch from New York; and Bacon Chow from Johns Hopkins, virtually all of the pioneers

15

in the field are still active in research, and most were present at the conference. It should also be noted that the field has generated more questions than answers and in being young will, it is hoped, have the vigor and time advantage to evolve solutions.

Historically, the study of nutrition, brain development, and behavior has followed the pattern of the classical trilogy in which a problem is recognized clinically; clinical and animal research are joined to provide information and understanding; and finally this new knowledge is applied to the resolution of the human situation.

My interest in the field was stimulated during the early 1950's with the discovery of the effects of a borderline deficiency of a single nutrient, vitamin B_6, on the neurochemical, neurophysiological, and clinical behavior of the human infant. By that time, Josef Brozek was already deeply involved in the field and, since 1941, had been examining the consequences of acute nutrient deficiency on adult human behavior. Geber and Dean in Africa had been following human populations for evidence of malnutrition and concurrent impairment of nervous system function, as had Rafael Ramos-Galván in Mexico, Joaquin Cravioto in Guatemala, and M. B. Stoch and P. M. Smythe in Africa.

By the 1960's, widening interest in human and animal research began to emerge. There was a dissertation on the subject at Cornell in 1962, and, during the 1963 meeting of the International Congress of Nutrition in Edinburgh, R. A. McCance and E. M. Widdowson not only were expressing interest in the changes in size of the pigs that they were affecting with malnutrition and then refeeding, but were also becoming concerned with their brain growth. John Dobbing was part of that scene, and a report on his excellent work since that time appears in chapter 4 below. At Cornell, Ricciuti was exploring the effects of malnutrition on cognitive development. In Guatemala, the Institute of Nutrition of Central America and Panama (INCAP) was expanding beyond the early interests of Cravioto into a major longitudinal study under Robert Klein.

In 1966 Richard Barnes published a paper on the subject, expressing his findings with his customary precaution so as not to be misinterpreted. In that year the field was dignified by being listed for a half-day session at the Hamburg meeting of the International Congress of Nutrition. In 1967 at the M.I.T. Conference on the subject many of the world's scholars from numerous disciplines expressed their views and suggested that solutions to the numerous problems would shortly be in hand. Unfortunately, this has not been the case, but the multifactorial nature of the effects of malnutrition has attracted the energies of scientists from a wide variety of disciplines who are currently exploring their separate avenues of research.

Among these investigators have been people like Myron Winick, who has put cellular hyperplasia and hypertrophy into proper perspective; Robert Zimmermann, who has been working with primates; Adolfo Chávez, who has been concerned with the stimulation of malnourished human infants; and Slávka Fraňková and Josef Lát, from Czechoslovakia, who have made significant contributions to our understanding of performance and behavior in the rat. Stephen Zamenhof and Edith van Marthens demonstrated that circumstances are much worse if malnutrition starts early in life, and, if the individual experiences prenatal and postnatal malnutrition, the situation is at its worst.

Various publications such as the *Journal of Nutrition* began to reflect this activity. The august Federation of American Societies of Experimental Biology held sessions on malnutrition and brain development and published the proceedings.

By 1969, Barnes had become very concerned with the experimental scene: nutritionists who had little background in the appropriate disciplines were doing behavioral and performance studies, while experimental psychologists were taking nutrition for granted as an insignificant variable in their studies. Barnes, therefore, convened a cross section of experts in the fields of experimental psychology and nutrition at the Battelle Institute in Seattle, and the resultant interaction between these two groups stimulated a great deal of new activity. The Prague meeting in 1969 of the International Congress of Nutrition included a number of sessions on malnutrition and brain development; a meeting held in England under Bacon Chow's guidance brought forth more new pieces of information to the field; in 1972, the International Congress of Nutrition in Mexico and, in 1975, the International Congress in Kyoto, Japan, held extensive sessions on malnutrition and behavior.

The year 1976, too, was replete with a series of specialized meetings on the subject: a conference was held in Cali, Colombia, that included discussion of data from the six major longitudinal human malnutrition studies in this hemisphere by representatives from the Rush-Susser group from the United States; the Cravioto-DeLicardi group from Mexico; the Chávez group in Mexico; the Klein group from Guatemala; the Mora-Herrera-Cremer group from Bogotá, Colombia; and the Sinisterra-McKay group from Colombia. In every one of these milestone meetings Barnes played a significant role either by his personal presence or through his influence on the research that had been undertaken.

Today, though we are moving forward rapidly, we have increasing need for the kinds of data that will be helpful in policy planning to cope with the interrelated problems of nutrition, brain development, and behavior in this country and throughout the world. At the present time, many of these decisions are being made arbitrarily, based on the meager information now available. It is hoped that future guidance will come from the new findings presented here.

Richard H. Barnes **2**

Reflections on the Study of Malnutrition and Mental Development

The influence of nutritional status on behavior has been recognized for many years. One has only to skim through the masterful review of this subject published by Josef Brozek and his colleague Gilbert Vaes in 1961 titled "Experimental investigations on the effects of dietary deficiencies on animal and human behavior"[3] to realize that the subject has attracted attention since the early years of this century. It is then somewhat surprising that organized research dealing with the problem of behavior and intellectual development in children suffering from the devastating and world-wide scourge of protein-calorie malnutrition (PCM) was not undertaken until about 1955. To be sure, observant clinicians had noted behavioral abnormalities in malnourished children, but such observations apparently had little effect in stimulating research in this area. For example, Julio Meneghello in 1949 published a report in which he pointed out that psychological changes noted in hospitalized malnourished children were not simply a response to hospitalization, since the changes were already apparent when the children were admitted.

Even though by 1955 it was generally being recognized that severe protein-calorie malnutrition, which up to this time had been called protein malnutrition, was associated with abnormal behavior, no serious thought appears to have been given either to possible long-lasting effects of malnutrition or to lack of social or sensory stimulation. In fact, the following quote from D. B. Jelliffe's book *Infant Nutrition in the Subtropics and Tropics*, published in 1955,[16] suggests this thought:

A point of interest that has been raised recently is the fact that some of the mental features seen in kwashiorkor resemble those due to "maternal deprivation," occurring, for example, in motherless infants in orphanages. The clinical picture of this condition has been fully described by Bowlby in his excellent monograph. Relevant features appear to include misery, refusal of food, apathy, and withdrawal. These also occur in kwashiorkor, when, apart from the nutritional deficiencies of the weaning period, the infant has also recently experienced the psychological shock of sudden displacement from the breast, often after a very prolonged period of breast-feeding. While to the writer it seems very probable that this situation produces psychological trauma, which certainly requires more investigation, the mental features of kwashiorkor seem to become reversed too rapidly with suitable protein treatment, especially with skimmed milk, to be explicable solely on a psychological basis.

In 1955 M. B. Stoch and P. M. Smythe initiated their long-term longitudinal study upon the hypothesis "that undernutrition during infancy may result in failure of the brain to achieve its full potential size and it is not unreasonable to suppose that this may also predispose to inhibition of optimum intellectual and personality development."[21] This study involved the selection of two groups of children, approximately 10 months to 2 years of age, one group undernourished, the other in good nutritional health. Both groups were from a low socioeconomic population in Cape Town, South Africa. Measurements of growth, head circumference, and IQ's have been made, and a follow-up of these subjects is still continuing.

In the light of present-day knowledge, observations in a 1919 publication by Smiley Blanton[2] are remarkable in that they predate general acceptance of one of the most important conclusions concerning malnutrition and mental development by more than fifty years. Blanton, a medical officer in the U.S. Army, was assigned to study the physical changes occurring in the school children of Trier, Germany, as a result of malnutrition caused by war conditions. He encountered so many complaints from teachers concerning mental deterioration of the children as shown in poor school work that it was decided to supplement the physical examination by a psychiatric study to determine just what the conditions were. Several thousand children had been forced to subsist for three years upon a rigid and inadequate diet. From this population, 6,500 children of the Volksschulen in Trier between five and one-half and fourteen years of age were examined. Among a number of other conclusions drawn from this study the following are of general interest in reflecting interpretations made in the early part of the twentieth century as to the effect of malnutrition on mental development.

The specific changes noted in the children caused by malnutrition are: (a) a lack of nervous and physical energy; (b) inattention during school hours; (c) poor and slow comprehension for school tasks; (d) poor memory for school work; (e) a general nervous restlessness while in school.

Children of good nervous stock of superior or good average intelligence can withstand malnutrition of even a serious degree extending over more than two years without any impairment of the intelligence or any definite emotional change; a lack of nervous energy is about all the change that occurs. Children of poor nervous stock with poor or inferior intelligence suffer a general and sometimes a permanent lowering of the whole intelligence level from even a moderate degree of malnutrition. But not more than five per cent of the total school population have suffered injury to the nervous system such as to affect the intelligence permanently.

It is interesting to reflect on observations, deductions, and conclusions drawn by scientists long before the additional facts have made possible a more accurate interpretation of their scientific research. For example, Blanton's first five conclusions as to the effects of malnutrition certainly coincide with currently accepted behavioral changes associated with malnutrition. However, the most impressive observation and deduction was the association of permanence of retarded intelligence with a low level of intelligence of the parents. Today we might extend this deduction to conclude that permanence may be associated with a low level of stimulation provided by parents of lower general intellectual development.

In the last 1950's Joaquin Cravioto and his collaborators published preliminary reports of some of their work that for the first time showed that severe PCM might result in long-lasting impairment in psychological development.[19] In a more formal report of these observations[8] published in 1963, evidence was presented by this group that malnourished preschool-age children exhibited decreased mental age and that with increasing chronological age the gap between mental age and chronological age increased. However, children admitted to the hospital showed increasing mental age so that the gap with chronological age decreased except for children admitted under 6 months of age in whom there was no such improvement. In this same publication Cravioto

Richard H. Barnes

commented in a particularly enlightened manner as follows:

> Any attempt to measure the influence of nutrition on mental performance must consider of necessity the role played by parental factors, such as maternal concern with intellectual development, maternal deprivation and parental level of intelligence. The relative weightings to be given to parental factors depend upon a series of other environmental conditions. Fo young children in preindustrialized countries food consumption and its consequence, nutritional status, is one of the most important.

Thus by 1960 there had been a general recognition that PCM caused psychological changes to develop in infants and young children, and there was an initiation of a few longitudinal studies with preliminary evidence of long-lasting retardation in certain measures of behavioral development, particularly in infants with PCM when less than 6 months of age.

In retrospect it is puzzling that so much evidence had accumulated by the 1960's, which, if put together, showed clearly that general malnutrition, in many cases partial starvation, caused behavioral changes that interfered with intellectual development, yet so few studies in either children or experimental animals had been carried out.

Since 1920 it had been recognized that undernutrition imposed during early postnatal life in the rat resulted in permanent growth stunting, not only of total body weight, but also of brain weight.[15] John Cowley and R. D. Griesel in 1959 had published results showing that a relatively small decrease in protein content of a diet fed to weanling female rats slightly reduced their growth but had no effect upon their learning performance in a Hebb-Williams maze. However, when these females were bred and their progeny were fed the maternal low-protein diet, their performance in maze learning was inferior to well-fed controls, thus showing a generational enhancement effect of malnutrition upon learning behavior.[5] Research was extended to a second generation, and results were published in 1963.[6] The second generation low-protein rats were nutritionally rehabilitated and continued to show learning deficits, thus illustrating for the first time that the effects of malnutrition were not only long-lasting, but that they could carry over a generation that was well fed.[7]

Even though the Cowley and Griesel studies showed this amazing generational effect of mild protein deficiency, the extensive research effort that we see in the malnutrition-behavior arena

22

today required something more to really set it in motion. In my opinion this impetus was provided by the biochemists working on early malnutrition and brain development. The initial studies of John Dobbing and his colleagues, published in 1964, showed an inhibition of brain myelination by PCM imposed upon rats during a vulnerable period in their early development.[9, 10] Furthermore, an outstanding contribution by Myron Winick and Adele Noble[22] showed that restriction of food intake from birth to 21 days of age in the rat resulted in a decrease in brain DNA indicative of a decreased number of cells in the brain and that this deficit remained even though the animals were nutritionally rehabilitated. These studies provided biological evidence of brain damage, which in the minds of many was causally associated with the evidence of retarded intellectual development in children and with measurements showing poor learning performance in early malnourished animals. This provocative interpretation of altered brain development causing retarded mental development in malnourished children carried the stigma that retarded mental development in early-malnourished children was permanent, and that correcting the nutritional condition could have little effect upon intellectual development. The specter of millions of infants and young children relegated to a life of the mentally retarded as a result of malnutrition helped immeasurably in promoting the importance of good nutritional care of children and the development of special food programs that have helped combat malnutrition. Nevertheless, this interpretation of a causal relationship of so-called "brain damage" and retardation of behavioral and intellectual development had to be modified when it was recognized that social and environmental stimulation of malnourished animals held the potential for altering or even obliterating the behavioral consequences of the malnutrition. Demonstration of this remarkable effect of the interaction of nutrition and environment was spearheaded by Slávka Fraňková. Her results on behavioral modification produced by handling malnourished rat pups were presented at the 1967 M.I.T. Conference on Malnutrition, Learning, and Behavior.[12]

Relatively recent publications have resulted from general awareness of this very important interaction phenomenon. Among these have been additional animal studies confirming and extending information relating to specific behavior characteristics modified by stimulation [13, 17] and studies in children showing that early malnutrition occurring in families of normal educational, social, and economic background did not result in any long-lasting impairment of intellectual development of the child.[18,20] This background information together with a general lack of evidence of retarded intellectual development in mild to moderate malnourished children has led to a current conclusion that is clearly stated in a World Health Organization (WHO) summary of the 1974 symposium on "Early Malnutrition and Mental Development" of the Swedish Nutrition Foundation.

The most important conclusion that can be drawn from the discussions at both the symposium and the workshop was that, in spite of the widely held and widely publicized opinion that malnutrition in early life jeopardizes mental development, the evidence to support this opinion—especially that from studies conducted in man—is scanty. Furthermore, most of the work has been carried out on children suffering from extreme degrees of malnutrition and there is practically no evidence of a relationship between the much commoner mild and moderate forms of malnutrition and mental retardation. What seems probable is that there is an interaction between malnutrition and other environmental factors, especially social stimulation, and that the child's ultimate intellectual status is the resultant of this interaction.[1]

Not always do the interpretations of scientists hold true over the years. Additional data frequently modify these interpretations. Thus at the meeting at Cornell University held in November 1975, we compared observations that have been reported from longitudinal studies conducted in Mexico and Guatemala with the conclusions drawn from the Swedish Nutrition Foundation Symposium held in 1974. Current results do show clearly that mild-to-moderate malnutrition in children does jeopardize mental development. At the same time supportive evidence of the importance of stimulation in modifying the damaging effects of malnutrition has also been presented. With reference to these latter conclusions one cannot help but wonder, were Blanton with us today, if he would respond—"I told you so."

It takes a few years for new scientific information to infiltrate ongoing research programs when such information is outside the mainstream of primary research interest. Neurophysiologists and biochemists have been looking at the effects of either malnutrition or stimulation on parameters that define their specific research interest. It would appear that the most exciting and important advances will be made by these scientists when they start to unravel the neurological complexities of the interactions of nutritional status and stimulation. We have made a start in this direction and have recently reported that the change in activity of cholinergic enzymes in the brain that takes place when rats are exposed to early malnutrition is abolished when rat pups during the suckling period are exposed to stimulation in the form of handling.[11] It is hoped that this area will become a part of the steep slope of the sigmoidal growth curve that we are now experiencing in studies relating to malnutrition and mental development.

Another approach in the neurophysiological area that has been developing with increasing speed is the electroencephalographic measurement of evoked responses. This direction of study of early malnutrition has been pioneered and nurtured through recent years by David Coursin, and I am sure we will hear much more along this line of study in the near future.

An area of research utilizing the experimental animal model of PCM that has been written and talked about, but sadly neglected, is the use of this model to study the action of pharmacologic agents. There is, of course, the potential for certain drugs to modify in a beneficial way the deleterious effects of malnutrition on mental development. Fránková has been a pioneer in this area of study and even though some encouraging results have been obtained,[14] the surface has only been scratched. Also of potential importance is the use of the PCM animal as a model for such behaviors as elevated emotionality under aversive situations, decreased attention span, decreased memory, apathy to novel objects in the environment and other characteristics. These are seen not only in human PCM or experimental animal PCM where they can be readily duplicated, but also in other mental disorders in man. This should offer the psychopharmacologist a new dimension in his search for agents that modify behavior.

The study of early malnutrition and mental development in experimental animals provides a dramatic illustration of the multidisciplinary nature of nutrition research and points out the need for collaborative research groups involving nutrition scientists, behavior scientists, biochemists, neurochemists, psychopharmacologists, and many other scientific specialties. It will be extremely hazardous for the individual, regardless of the field of his scientific expertise, to "go it alone" in the investigation of many of the complex problems of early malnutrition. Furthermore, mak-

Richard H. Barnes

ing the study of early malnutrition even more exciting is the fact that long-lasting or permanent effects also have been noted in energy, protein, fat, and carbohydrate metabolism as well as many changes in endocrine function. The most recently discovered biological malfunctioning due to early malnutrition is depressed antibody formation in early malnourished rats. This impairment was found to continue through two filial generations of offspring of malnourished dams.[4] Surely, we have only begun to uncover and study the many facets of this exciting subject.

Reference

1. Anonymous. *W.H.O. Chronicle* 28: 95, 1974.
2. Blanton, S. Mental and nervous changes in children of the Volksschulen of Trier, Germany, caused by malnutrition. *Mental Hygiene* 3: 343, 1919.
3. Brozek, J., and G. Vaes. Experimental investigations on effects of dietary deficiency on animal and human behavior. *Vitam. Hormones* 19: 43, 1961.
4. Chandra, R. K. Antibody formation in first and second generation offspring of nutritionally deprived rats. *Science* 190: 289, 1975.
5. Cowley, J. J. and R. D. Griesel. Some effects of a low protein diet on a first filial generation of white rats. *J. Genet. Psychol.* 95: 187, 1959.
6. Cowley, J. J., and R. D. Griesel. The development of second-generation low protein rats. *J. Genet. Psychol.* 103: 233, 1963.
7. Cowley, J. J., and R. D. Griesel. The effect on growth and behaviour of rehabilitating first and second generation low protein rats. *Anim. Behav.* 14: 506, 1966.
8. Cravioto, J. Application of newer knowledge of nutrition on physical and mental growth and development. *Am. J. Pub. Health* 53: 1803, 1963.
9. Davison, A. N., and J. Dobbing. Myelination as a vulnerable period in brain development. *Brit. Med. Bull.* 22: 40, 1966.
10. Dobbing, J. The influence of early nutrition on the development and myelination of the brain. *Proc. Roy. Soc. Biol.* 159: 503, 1964.
11. Eckhert, C. D., D. A. Levitsky, and R. H. Barnes. Postnatal stimulation: The effects on cholinergic enzyme activity in undernourished rats. *Proc. Soc. Expl. Biol. Med.* 149: 860, 1975.
12. Fraňková, S. Nutritional and psychological factors in the development of spontaneous behavior in the rat. In *Malnutrition, Learning, and Behavior,* N. S. Scrimshaw and J. E. Gordon, eds., M.I.T. Press, Cambridge, Mass., 1968.
13. Fraňková, S. Interaction between early malnutrition and stimulation in animals. In J. Cravioto, L. Hambraeus, and B. Vahlquist, eds., *Early Malnutrition and Mental Development: Symp. Swedish Nutr. Found.,* XII, Almquist and Wiksell, Uppsala, 1974.

14. Franková, S., and O. Benesova. Effect of pyrithioxine (encephabol) on growth and exploratory behavior of rats malnourished in early life. *Psychopharmacologia* (Berlin) 28: 63, 1973.
15. Jackson, C. M., and A. C. Stewart. The effects of inanition in the young upon ultimate size of the body and of various organs in the albino rat. *J. Exp. Zool.* 30: 97, 1920.
16. Jelliffe, D. B. *Infant Nutrition in the Subtropics and Tropics.* *W.H.O.* Geneva, 1955.
17. Levitsky, D. A., and R. H. Barnes. Nutritional and environmental interactions in behavioral development of the rat: Long-term effects. *Science* 176: 68, 1972.
18. Lloyd-Still, J. D., I. Hurwitz, P. H. Wolff, and H. Shwachman. Intellectual development after severe malnutrition in infancy. *Pediatrics* 54: 306, 1974.
19. Robles, B., R. Ramos-Galvan, and J. Cravioto. Evaluation of the behavior of the child with advanced malnutrition and its modification during recovery. (Preliminary report in Spanish.) *Bol. Med. Hosp. Infant* (Mexico) 16: 317, 1959.
20. Stein, Z., M. Susser, G. Saenger, and F. Marolla. *Famine and Human Development: The Dutch Hunger Winter.* Oxford University Press, New York, 1975.
21. Stoch, M. B., and P. M. Smythe. Does undernutrition during infancy inhibit brain growth and subsequent intellectual development? *Arch. Dis. Child.* 38: 548, 1963.
22. Winick, M., and A. Noble. Cellular response in rats during malnutrition at various ages. *J. Nutr.* 89: 300, 1966.

Malnutrition, Environment, and Child Development

Man is first of all a biological species and, as such, has ways and means that do not differ from those of any other species of life. He is primarily motivated to search for a place where his favorite food is abundant, eat as much as possible of that food, and produce as many of his strain as possible, so that they can go and search for their food, eat what they can, and produce a new series of off-spring that will then repeat the cycle.

One day, for reasons not well known to us, man changed, asked for a companion and eventually became a social as well as a biological species. As a social species, he invented culture and technology. It is only recently that man has become concerned about the fate of his species, and particularly about the future of his children. He has been trying to understand why children grow and has learned that there are two groups of children in this world, some of whom, the minority, are born under good care and surroundings, receive good stimulation, and are able to profit from the culture of their ancestors; others, the vast majority, are born into conditions that cannot be called human in the social sense. Children from the second group are made to assume adult roles at too early an age. They lack protection, stimulation, and good nutrition. They are almost totally deprived of the advantages enjoyed by the minority.

My colleagues and I have been concerned for a number of years with the effect of the environment and, within the environment, the effect of nutrition on children, especially on their mental and social development. We started our work in a rural Mexican village. We observed a significant correlation between the developmental age of these children and their theoretical height for age: the greater the height of the children, up to a point, the better their developmental quotient, and the more they were retarded in height, the greater the chance of their having a low developmental quotient.

This held true for populations not only in northern Mexico, but also in central Mexico, the southern part of Mexico, Guatemala, Salvador, Costa Rica, Panama, Nigeria, and Ghana. It can be shown that in rural areas the distribution of developmental quotients of children from lower socioeconomic levels, particularly older children, is clearly different from that of children from a better socioeconomic class. The children from a good socioeconomic class have scores similar to those of a good socioeconomic class in industrialized countries in both physical growth and developmental level, whereas those from lower socioeconomic levels in rural villages who have retarded physical growth display lower rates of cognitive development. So our first question was whether the retarded mental and social development was related to retarded physical growth. We conducted, then, a series of cross-sectional studies attempting to answer that question.

First, we looked for any biochemical lesion that may have been caused by the factors we believed to be associated with the poorer growth rate of these children. We conducted studies of amino acids. In the children admitted to a hospital with severe malnutrition, the ratios of phenylalanine to tyrosine, and of tyrosine to cysteine were comparable to the ratios one observes in phenylketonuria. We thought that probably this was the reason for poorer cognitive development, but just 3 to 4 weeks after nutritional rehabilitation the blood changes would disappear: the children no longer showed any signs of the biochemical lesion, yet they continued to show signs of delayed cognitive development.

We took electroencephalograms of the children when they were severely malnourished and observed profound alterations. Yet after 3 or 4 months of recovery, there were still some abnormalities in the electroencephalograph.

When we studied the IQ's of children who had been malnourished when they were under 3 years of age and had had 2 years or more of recovery, we found twice as many of these children with IQ's below 70 as we did among their siblings who had not been severely malnourished. On the other hand, only 4 of the previously malnourished children had IQ's of 90 or more as compared to 10 of their well-nourished controls.

For a more sophisticated examination of cognitive development, we examined various forms of intersensory integration by testing the ability of children to correlate information entering the brain from different sensory modalities. The development of visual-auditory integration, for example, is essential in order to learn to read. We observed significantly lower scores in visual-auditory integration in those children who had recovered from severe malnutrition when compared to their well-nourished siblings. The previously malnourished children were always behind at every age level until the age of 11.

Another kind of intersensory integration, visual-kinosthetic integration, is a prerequisite for learning to write. We again found that the children who were previously malnourished made more errors than their siblings who had never been severely malnourished.

Another aspect of cognitive development of children, known as transitivity, is the formation of mathematical concepts. Transitivity is the ability to reason that if A is greater than B, and B is greater than C, then A has to be greater than C. We observed that the percentage of children that perceived transitivity was greater in children of the upper social class showing good growth than among those of the lower social class whose development was characterized by poor growth.

When these data were replotted on cognitive performance as a function of height rather than age, little evidence was found of a functional relationship between height and measures of cognitive performance among children of the upper socioeconomic class. Among those of the lower socioeconomic class, on the other hand, increase in height was almost always accompanied by increase in performance. This strongly suggests that nutrition is a far greater limiting factor on growth and intellectual development in the lower socioeconomic group than in the upper socioeconomic class where genetics may be the primary determinant of height.

Malnutrition, however, does not occur in isolation. Even if you can demonstrate by cross-sectional studies that children who were malnourished performed at lower levels in a series of tests, had lower IQ's, and lacked the prerequisites for reading, writing, or formation of mathematical concepts, you have proved only one thing: that in those cases the low physical growth was accompanied by low mental performance.

Malnutrition is a very complex ecological phenomenon, and to describe it I would like to present the following paradigm. What happens in a society when technology is not applied in a systematic manner? One result is a "low purchasing power" for the individual. Low purchasing power means that a high proportion of an individual's time (and energy) must be spent on acquiring the bare necessities of life. Consequently, not enough time, money, and effort are available for investment in sanitation, and primitive concepts of health and disease persist.

The persistence is illustrated in the traditional ways of feeding children. In the culture of survival, the mother (through many generations) has acquired the wisdom of the scientist. The scientist reasons that if A is present when B is present, and A is absent when B is absent, then the probability of a causal relationship between A and B is a high one. A mother in such circumstances reasons that if diarrhea appears when food is given, and diarrhea disappears when food is taken away, then there must be a causal relationship between the two. There is a causal relationship, but the mother does not understand because she has only a primitive concept of health. She does not know about pathogenic bacteria, and she is unaware that it is not the food but the contamination of the food that produces the diarrhea. So to her the best thing to do is to suppress food from the diet of the children, and in so doing she suppresses in general all those foods which are the best culture media for pathogens. She is absolutely right that this is the way to preserve life. So she will persist in the traditional distribution of food and reduce food intake in the sick child.

We know that in low-purchasing-power societies there will be early school leaving; there will be illiteracy; there will be less opportunity to receive adequate information. This will perpetuate the nonsystematic approach to society and consequently the persistence of primitive concepts. This was the reason why extension services were invented.

Extension services were intended to give school-age children who were no longer in the school some knowledge of better techniques for cultivation and production of food. Girls were taught how to raise better children, how to give better child care, and something about home management.

In societies where children leave school at an early age, two populations are created: one that remains in school, and one that goes to work and increases purchasing power. When in these societies a child of school age gets to be a provider, he becomes automatically an adult, in a sense. One of the things adults do is get married. He marries, of course, somebody who has left school, so the probability of a mating of two uneducated or barely educated persons is tremendously increased. The marriage is consummated at a very early age, resulting in an increased probability of a large family, closely spaced children, and inadequate child care. This cycle will probably be repeated over again, not because of a lack of food alone, but because of all of the inadequacies of the environment, primarily insufficient resources to permit education.

Because of this situation, you have a persistence of primitive health concepts and little knowledge of nutrition. There will be inadequate sanitary conditions, a lack of personal cleanliness which may lead to infections, and inadequate care of the child, with three probable consequences: (1) the reduction of food intake in the child; (2) the production of catabolism in the individual; and (3) an increased percentage of energy expenditure for health services merely in terms of time. The mother has to invest more time in taking care of a sick child than a well child, and this will result in a lower purchasing power for the family. When one tries to judge the effects of malnutrition on the development of the child, each one of these consequences is in itself adequate enough to produce a negative impact on the development of both mental and social competence in the child.

If one wants to pursue this further, one must study all the different variables together. In order to accomplish this we began an ecologic study in a community where malnutrition was highly prevalent. In such a community we found up to 9 percent of third-degree malnutrition and up to 21 percent of mild-to-moderate malnutrition in children of ages between 2 and 3 years. We performed a study with three aims in mind. The first was to learn something about the effect of malnutrition on semantic growth and mental development and learning. The second was to learn the interactions among nutritional practice, infectious disease, family circumstances, social variables, and the process of growth and development. Finally, the third aim was to learn about the influences of those social, economic, and family circumstances on the development of malnutrition.

We took a community of 7,000 people, 3,500 children below the age of 15 years, and collected data on all the deliveries that occurred within one calendar year. Out of those 300 or so deliveries there were 22 cases of severe malnutrition. The infant mortality expected in the first year of life was 96 per 1,000 live births. During our stay it was reduced to 37 per 1,000 live births. One can lower the mortality by providing community services. One cannot influence the morbidity because community medicine has nothing to do with morbidity. It saves lives but it doesn't solve problems.

Our sample contained 22 cases of malnutrition, 15 of kwashiorkor, and 7 of marasmus. I would like to point out three things in regard to these longitudinal studies. First, the growth curves of malnourished and nonmalnourished children were alike until about 12 months of age, when cases of malnutrition first became apparent. Second, there was no difference in language development until the time of the appearance of malnutrition, at which point differences in language development began to appear. The language development of those children with malnutrition was significantly slower from 12 months on than that of the other group of children who were never malnourished. Even at 3 years of age, when all children suffering from malnutrition had recovered, a very large difference in language development was still apparent.

Malnutrition also delays the formation of concepts in children. The difference in rate of concept formation became apparent at approximately 26 months of age. We studied primarily the formation of bipolar concepts. Some examples of our bipolar concepts are: black and white, dry and wet, full and empty, inside and outside, above and below, big and small, slow and fast. One can demonstrate that this process is developmental in nature, that is, as age advances the number of concepts present in the child also advances. We presented to the child a series of pairs of objects that were exactly the same in form, in shape, in consistency, but they differed in the two poles—for example, one was black and the other was white. After several examples, we tested to see if the child could designate the two poles. Those children with malnutrition or who had been rehabilitated from malnutrition after 42 months of age all exhibited fewer concepts than their well-nourished controls. It is important to point out that after an initial delay in the development of bipolar concept, development proceeded at a rate comparable to controls. We call this delayed development, not arrested development. Even at 46 months of age the difference in the development of bipolar concepts was still quite striking, the malnourished children always lagging behind the controls.

These malnourished children differed from their controls qualitatively as well as quantitatively. We can assess not only how much the children score, but also the style of responding. We can ask a child to answer a question. He can respond by attempting to figure out the answer or by refusing to try to answer. In either case, he may be verbal or nonverbal. Among the previously malnourished children only half of the children responded to a task affirmatively, whereas 80 percent of the well-nourished children responded affirmatively. Only 6 out of 10 of the previously malnourished children responded verbally, whereas 8 out of the 10 well-nourished children responded verbally.

If we look at the manner in which a child verbalizes his refusal to answer, we find four different ways he can respond. He can express his refusal in terms of competence, a rationalization. For example, a child might say, "I cannot do it because I am very small." "I cannot do it because you have never taught me how to do it." "I cannot do it because I have not practiced." Second, a child just may give an indication, "No, I won't do it." Alternatively, the child may behave in terms of substitution: "I want to go to my mother." "Take me to the wash room." "Give me the dolls." "I prefer to walk with the dolls." Anything, except doing what is demanded of him, like a good student. Finally, the child may request aid, which means "do it for me." Now, when one contrasts the two groups, a clear difference emerges in the style of refusing. The survivors of malnutrition mainly requested aid and used substitute behaviors in refusing to work on the problem. The controls refused mainly because they felt a lack of competence. They solicited very little aid and used very few substitutions.

Another way to explore behavior, particularly social behavior, is to explore if the child believes that his behavior influences others' behavior. We may present a picture of a father and tell the child that the father is very happy. We ask the child, "If you were his child why would the father be happy? Is he happy because you are doing your best, or because the father had an easy day?" If the child answers that the father is happy because the father had an easy day, we interpret it as indicating that the child's behavior doesn't influence others. If the child answers that the father is happy because he is doing his best, we interpret this as indicating that the child does believe his behavior influences others. We give the child a series of these pictures and obtain a profile of our two groups. Of those children who were survivors of malnutrition only 4 out of 10 believed their behavior influenced others, whereas 8 out of 10 controls indicated such. Therefore, it is not only the quantitative aspect of behavior which differs, but behavior we can ascribe to the socialistic aspects. Malnutrition not only disrupts the cognitive development quantitatively, but also alters the behavior qualitatively by producing different response styles and perhaps self-perceptions.

We stated earlier that malnutrition does not appear in isolation but is part of the total ecology of poverty. We compared some of the characteristics of the parents of malnourished children to those of parents of well-nourished children, matched for size and performance at birth. There was no statistical difference in mother's age, father's age, height and weight of both parents, or the parity of the mother. There also was no difference in family size, personality, age of previously born children, or proportion of nuclei extended family. More surprising, there was no statistical difference in the annual income per capita, the percentage of total expenses that were devoted to food procurement, or the presence of sanitary facilities in the household. No differences were found in the personal cleanliness of the mother, the personal cleanliness of the father, change in formal education from grandmother to mother. There was no difference in proportion of literate to illiterate mothers.

There were, however, clear differences between the two groups. Fifty percent of the mothers of malnourished children listened regularly to the radio, while about 75 percent of the mothers of well-nourished children did. There was a question of interpretation. When you have 20 comparisons and one of these comparisons is significant, it is possible that this results in a statistical error. In 1963 in a study in Guatemala we found that those children with better gains in weight during the first semester of life also had a higher percentage of mothers who listened regularly to the radio and a higher percentage of mothers who would speak Spanish to their children instead of their local dialect. Thus, we do not believe that we are dealing with a statistical error, but are in fact dealing with a different kind of mother.

To test this possibility we undertook a study of home stimulations. We monitored the level of home stimulation of the child every month from the beginning of life, using the instrument devised by Caldwell.[1] This inventory covered nine areas of stimulation that are supposed to foster cognition, growth, and development. An example of an item in this inventory assesses whether a family usually converses freely at meals, and, if so, whether the child participates. Another item asks if the parents occasionally sing to the child or sing in the presence of the child. Another assesses whether the parents encourage the child to relate his experiences or take the time to listen to him relate his experiences.

At 6 months of age we found the homes of all the children which later developed malnutrition rated no more than 36 points in home stimulation. It must be emphasized that at this point in time only 1 child was observed to be malnourished. The rest were not malnourished at the time of observation, and we had no idea which child would later become malnourished. None of the control children, who did not develop malnutrition, had scores lower than 32. Even after the bout with malnutrition, the homes of the malnourished children continued to rate less "stimulation" than the homes of the well-nourished children. None of the controls scored less than 100; one-half of the malnourished children scored less than 90. Thus, there was less home stimulation before and after the period of malnutrition in comparison with homes in which the children did not develop malnutrition.

Another way to assess the environment of the child is to analyze the child's interrelationships. We accomplished this by studying the mother-child interactions in the presence of a psychologist. We observed the child at the end of the first month of life. When the child who later became malnourished was performing easily on the tests the mother reacted with complete passivity, minimal reaction, acceptance without question. On the other hand, most mothers of children who later did not develop malnutrition watched with pride and admiration at seeing their children performing adequately. Only 2 out of the 10 children whose mothers demonstrated this characteristic later developed malnutrition. As a result of a whole series of observations, this effect seemed quite repeatable. The mothers of children who later became malnourished showed significantly less responsiveness and pride than the mothers of children who avoided malnutrition.

If the level of stimulation and the responsiveness of the children are important to the development of the child, then one should be able to influence the course of recovery from malnutrition with the addition of these variables to the normal medical treatment of malnutrition. We have just begun to add stimulation and mother responsiveness as variables in the treatment of children who were malnourished below the age of 6 months. We trained the caretakers in giving the children systematic stimulation. These children recovered their cognitive deficits much faster than children who recovered without systematic stimulation.

Thus, we are able to pull out these important variables in the ecology of malnutrition: level of home stimulation, intellectual performance, malnutrition, and development of bipolar concepts. Let us look at the interrelationship of these factors. Let us use height as an indicator of malnutrition and bipolar concept formats as a measure of intellectual performance. Height correlated positively with bipolar concept information at the level of .26, home stimulation at the level of .20, and intellectual performance at the level of .67, all of which were highly significant. All of these variables were correlated and were then subjected to partial correlation analysis. The relationship between body height and intellectual performance was not affected by the number of bipolar concepts. However, the correlation between body height and number of bipolar concepts disappeared when one controlled for intellectual performance. This means that the relationship between body height and bipolar concepts is not a direct one, but is related through intellectual performance.

Moreover, when one held constant the number of bipolar concepts, the correlation between home stimulation and intellectual performance disappeared. Similarly, when one partialled out the level of intellectual performance, the relationship between home stimulation and number of bipolar concepts disappeared. Thus, the relationship between home stimulation and language development, as measured by bipolar concepts, is not a direct one, but is related through intellectual performance.

Finally, the relationship between body height and home stimulation also seemed to relate through intellectual performance. The correlation disappeared when level of intellectual performance was partialled out.

We interpret these findings as meaning that malnutrition, as indicated by body height, influences the learning of language through its effect on general intellectual performance. Home stimulation also affected the learning of language but also through the fostering of intellectual achievement. Thus, both malnutrition and home stimulation affected learning through a common mechanism, intellectual performance. It is important to note that the results of several of the animal studies pointed to the same conclusion—that the behavioral effects of malnutrition were very dependent upon environmental stimulation.

The study of the ecology of malnutrition has clearly shown

many interacting factors which affect the cognitive development of the child. Man has the ability and the capacity to alter those aspects which limit the malnourished child's potential. What is needed is the desire and then commitment to make those changes.

Reference

1. Caldwell, B., J. Heider, and B. Kaplan. The inventory of home stimulation. Paper presented at the meeting of the American Psychological Association, New York, 1966. (Available from Center for Early Development and Education, University of Arkansas at Little Rock, Little Rock, Arkansas 72204.)

PART II

MALNUTRITION AND
THE CENTRAL NERVOUS SYSTEM

John Dobbing **4**

Malnutrition and the Developing Brain: A Critical Review

Introduction

The time has come, I believe, to stand back a little and measure our knowledge and understanding of the part early undernutrition may play in reducing human intellectual capacity. Thus my presentation here will be concerned with concepts and generalities rather than new data.

A very respectable body of scientific thought holds that conjecture, speculation, and philosophy are of such small consequence compared with hard fact, experimentally or observationally ascertained, that only the latter is worthy of serious attention. Too many people are said to sit about in comfortable chairs dreaming up profound hypotheses without subjecting them to the inconvenience of reconciliation with the facts. Unfortunately there is one kind of subject which even the narrow, hardened scientist is driven to treating in this rather broader way. When the magnitude of a subject is so enormous, and compounded of such a large number of inseparably interacting variables, the majority of which are not even identifiable, let alone measured, the strictly factual approach may eventually let us down because the ascertainable facts are too tiny a proportion of the whole to be themselves of dominating significance; and it may well be that our own is one such subject. This is not, of course, to underrate the imperative need for hard results. It is merely a plea to have them considered occasionally in a wider, more realistic, more meaningful, and more lifelike setting.

John Dobbing

The Nature of the Question

My own position starts with very vague assumptions: that individuals are endowed with a certain potential for their intellectual achievement; that no one, however advantaged, ever completely achieves that potential; that most people in the world fall very far short of it; that the mismatch between potential and actual achievement is imposed by environmental disadvantage, mostly during development; and that it is our business here to assess to what extent undernutrition at any developmental stage, amidst a host of other interacting nonnutritional disadvantages, may play a part in restricting ultimate intellectual achievement.

All this, like so much of real life, is quite banal. It is also unscientific, in the sense that few, if any, of the terms can be satisfactorily defined or measured, and the hypothesis can probably never be properly tested. For me, however, this apparently vague concept is the yardstick by which the design of all investigations in this inquiry, as well as all results, must ultimately be measured.

We have to live, after all, in a jungle of similarly woolly concepts. What, for example, do the opposition mean when they ask (with all the appearance of precision), "Does infant or early malnutrition cause permanent mental retardation (or brain damage)"? There is no single term in this commonly formulated question which, when defined, does not restrict it to the point of destroying its usefulness. What do they mean by "infant or early"? For it is clear that unless the period of life be better defined for its vulnerability, we will be left with the earth-shattering conclusion that *we should feed children*. For practical social purposes, one of the few useful topics for investigation is whether there are stages of development which are more vulnerable than others. If there are, we may have to find ways of distributing our scarce resources to those priority groups. What does the question mean by "malnutrition"? The words "nutritional state" still elude meaningful definition. Are we to measure the quantity and quality of what goes in, and if so, for what period of life and for how long? If specific components of the diet, as broadly described as protein, or as finely described as folic acid, are indeed critical in this context (and my hunch is that they are not) we shall have to formulate the question a great deal more closely, and this may well destroy its applicability to humans.

When the question says "cause" (does malnutrition *cause* permanent mental retardation?), do we really mean it in the sense that the tubercle bacillus causes tuberculosis? (Actually it doesn't. Most of us can show lesions of our own caused by the tubercle bacillus, but few of us have suffered from tuberculosis.)

What do we mean by "permanent"? Do we mean a 5-year, a 10-year, or a 70-year follow up?

And finally, what do we mean by mental retardation? The term mental retardation in my language (and it certainly used to be mine) implies necessary connotations of severity and pathology. If someone has an intelligence quotient of 120, or of 97, when it might have been of 125 of 105, I do not call that mental retardation. Still less would I say that very large numbers of individuals in underprivileged communities are mentally retarded or *brain damaged*. Similarly, the clinical term "brain damage" means what it says. A part of the brain must have been destroyed focally. A child with Down's syndrome is not brain damaged, but he *is* mentally retarded, often very severely. "Mental retardation" and "brain damage" should be restricted to a narrower definition of the crudely pathological. And in case you regard this as yet another purely semantic discussion on the uses of my own language, let me remind you that neither the homes for dreadfully handicapped children nor the starved communities of preindustrial societies are occupied by cases of nutritionally induced mental retardation. Unless we accept that we are talking of the paranormal, or restrictions within the normal variance, we will be misled, as certain eminent epidemiologists have already been, into researching the incidence of Mongolism in such places as famine-stricken Bangladesh. Neither Mongolism, nor kernicterus, nor phenylketonuria, nor cerebral palsy is (for example) the Biafrans' most pressing problem even in the long term, and that is not just because the severely afflicted will have selectively died. Nor is there an epidemic of Wernicke's encephalopathy in the undernourished world.

Thus the question "Does early malnutrition cause permanent mental retardation?" is not only every bit as imprecise as my suggested alternative; it is also a great nonsense.

The Relative Importance of Nutrition

Whatever we think about the relative importance of early nutrition in shaping our individual destinies, it must surely be common ground now among all respectable persons of good will that our environment during our upbringing (rather than our genetic endowment) exerts an overwhelming influence on our ultimate personality and achievement. Our nutrition is merely a part of our developing environment, and our task is therefore to assess what relative size of influence developmental undernutrition may have on man's most distinctive attribute: his intellectual achievement.

Now if the multitude of environmental influences on our individual destinies were merely additive, we could set up a model along the lines of an algebraic sum. As it happens, it is a nonsense model because of the interactional nature of the real situation; but the algebraic sum idea is not a bad starting point. Let us suppose that there are 20 different environmental factors important to our intellectual development (there are probably nearer 20,000). Some of them come under group headings such as social class or the qualities of the home. These latter range from hygienic facilities to those which comprise "enrichment" of environmental stimulus. Another large number involve the emotional climate of the home, related to the maternal-infant relationship and all the other important relationships within the family. Another set of factors are known to relate to the geographical situation, for example "rural" or "urban," of the home. And then there are the educational facilities of the community and their quality; and then there is nutrition. It seems to me that if it were possible to break down all the other groups of factors into their individual components, no single one of them (not even nutrition) is likely to be quantitatively of enormous individual numerical importance. The algebraic sum model states that it is the sum of pluses and minuses among these factors which conditions the ultimate level of individual achievement. So it is a logical corollary that no single factor may be powerful in deciding the issue. In practical terms we have good reason to believe that a child may be quite seriously malnourished at all the important times, without any measurable effect on his subsequent performance, if he has accumulated enough counterbalancing pluses from his home or other nonnutritional environment.

Does this then mean that we cannot say that early nutrition is important to subsequent achievement? Of course not. Nutrition *is* important, but it probably need never be a dominant influence any more than any other single factor. Media men, and politicians do not like that kind of answer because it is too difficult for them. They much prefer to be able to identify a single factor which will cure the ills of the community. Nutrition, or even some single article of diet, is a sitting target for those who put simplicity of diagnosis before the real facts of life. This has a practical bearing on how we improve the intellectual outcome for the malnourished child or community. Certainly not by merely bringing in food. Successful measures must be attuned to the highly multifactorial nature of the problem, and that is much more difficult for the administrator.

These consequences of the algebraic sum idea are not, of course, quite as stark as we have portrayed them, due to the interactional nature of the various factors; but this enormously complicates the analysis.

Ancient Literature

Now I know there will be many who will say these things are so blindingly obvious that it is quite unnecessary to set them out. My evidence that this is not so could be drawn from prominent examples of quite recent research programs which I believe have been based on wrong initial concepts and have therefore not been very productive.

Unfortunately, the halting preambles to the presentation of such research too frequently rely on other than recent literature. There are very few papers published before 1970 that are sufficiently archival to stand such constantly repetitive citation except in the historical first chapter of a graduate student's thesis. One exception is the work of Winick and Noble.[14] Another is Widdowson and McCance.[13] Others in the human field are to be found in the writings of Cravioto[2] in the early sixties, and some others in the papers from Cornell. But it is high time that such old worthies as Stoch and Smythe (1963); Cabak and Najdanvic (1965); Platt, Stewart and Payne (1966); Dobbing and Widdowson (1965); and many others (like Dobbing 1964, 1968), cease to be quoted as incantations and seriously discussed. Modesty forbids a longer catalogue of outmoded references that are still widely quoted by people who have never even read them. Some were good enough papers in their day, but I am able to state that even their authors are now in many cases embarrassed at their continuing repetition.

Experimental Animals and Human Children

One whole chapter of investigation has inevitably been concerned with animal experiment, usually with the rat, but sometimes with pigs, dogs, guinea pigs, monkeys, and so forth. This is entirely healthy, and quite inevitable if we are to ask what effects undernutrition has on the physical development of the brain. The animal literature embraces a large number of pitfalls, but by far the largest is the proposal that an experimentally induced and demonstrable change in the physical brain is of functional importance, even when it is associated with concomitant behavioral changes in the same animal. We have clearly got to assume that behavioral changes have a physical basis. The error is to assume that the physical features we have described are the ones responsible.

It is, of course, quite respectable to research such changes, but if they are intended to illuminate the human condition, a series of frequently ignored criteria must absolutely be met. It is not that every animal preparation should mimic the human situation. Indeed many of the best experiments are highly contrived, and are designed to isolate one or another variable quite artificially. That is the main business of animal experiments, and those who grumble that rats are not like humans only demonstrate their own failure to grasp the point. However, the ultimate interpretation, extrapolating from rats to humans, is a cross-species extrapolation like any other, and the simple rules must be observed.

For example, a valid extrapolation must take into account the timing of the nutritional manipulation in relation to the developmental stages in human development which are equivalent to those in the experimental animal. It is not a matter of equivalent *ages*, but equivalent *stages*. Species differences in the timing of birth in relation to the common sequential pattern of brain growth are now well established. These make it a nonsense to compare the neonatal (or the fetal, or whatever else) rat with the neonatal guinea pig, or human, or pig, or monkey. The human newborn brain is at a quite different stage even from that of the monkey, and for all I know there may be yet more differences within the subhuman primate species themselves.

This point of view has been well rehearsed elsewhere.[7] Ignoring it has nowhere been more important and more misleading to humans than when pregnancy malnutrition has been researched in animals. The last one-third of pregnancy in any species is the time when maternal undernutrition results in retarded fetal growth and low birth weight for gestational age. This is as true for rats as for humans and, since the rat brain at this vulnerable time of its own species' pregnancy is passing through stages which occur at a correspondingly *invulnerable* time of human pregnancy (in early second trimester), the extrapolation from maternal rat nutrition to that in humans disobeys one of the golden rules of cross-species extrapolation and is misleading. It is also depressingly common in this context to ignore the rules relating to comparable *severity* of undernutrition across the species. It is claimed that maternal malnutrition in the rat can reduce rat birth weight by up to 20 or even 30 percent if it is severe enough. Now if the newborn rat brain has reached the stage of development attained by the mid-term human fetus, it will be necessary, before this preparation has any human significance, to show that the human brain can be reduced by maternal nutrition to a similar extent by about 20 or 25 weeks of gestation; to our knowledge this never happens.

The third rule, or "unity," which must be observed for valid cross-species extrapolation in this context is that of *duration*. The rat accomplishes in 6 or 7 weeks what humans take about 3 years to achieve. Thus the infliction of undernutrition or any other manipulation on a rat for a day is the human equivalent of a much longer period. This also applies to the lag periods which occur between the initiation of undernutrition or its cessation, and the effects becoming manifest.

If such rules as these are always observed, at least in our thinking if not in our experimental designs, species differences are no longer such inhibitors, and animal experiments become much more useful to those of us whose primary interest is in people. If the rules are not observed, our more perceptive critics will abandon us, and, what is worse, our masters will be seriously misled into evolving false measures to deal with our ailing world society.

Hyperplasia and Hypertrophy

As I have already implied, I believe the concept of hyperplasia being succeeded by hypertrophy during development of a tissue, and the bearing this has on catch-up potential following periods of adversity, is one of the most important ideas in growth and development to have been formulated this century. I also believe that its application to the developing brain has often been uncritical. Total brain cell number, as far as I know, is without any functional meaning, at least within the range of variation we are concerned with here. The architectural heterogeneity of the brain, compared with most other tissues, makes it necessary to specify which cells we are counting and *where.* Presumably neuronal deficits are more interesting to us than glial, and probably deficits in neuronal number which would be trivial in some brain regions would be catastrophic in others. When it comes to discussing hypertrophy in "brain cells," what do we mean? Are we talking about increasing oligodendroglial cytoplasm, neuronal cell bodies, or the cell mass which is represented in central nervous tissue by axons and the developing dendritic tree? If we postulate that only the *number* of cells is permanently affected and not their size, we are excluding the possible influence of the developing dendritic complexity and its synaptic connectivity (the number of synapses per neuron), both of which are apparently substantially and permanently reduced by undernutrition, and both of which appear in contemporary neurobiology to be much more significant to function than mere cell number. Any attempt to regionalize the biochemical analyses to take care of some of the whole organ heterogeneity renders the cell size index (protein per unit DNA) even less meaningful, since the smaller the region the more will its protein be derived from cells whose own DNA is not in the sample.

Super-rats

The proposal that people or animals can be made into supermen or "super-rats" by appropriately boosting the early nutritional or other environment, has no place in my thinking (a statement which has little enough bearing on whether it is true). I can understand the concept of "potential," for which we can strive with lesser or greater success, but I cannot understand the idea that the potential can be exceeded, except in science fiction. It can be shown, of course, that reducing the "normal" litter size of animals such as mice, rats, or rabbits results in larger animals whether the reduction be antenatal or immediately postnatal. Such larger animals have larger feet, larger livers, and larger brains. Perhaps it takes a larger brain to organize the physiological functions of larger bodies. But larger, for me, does not add up to "outstanding," a term which clearly implies intellectual brilliance, and I know of no evidence that relates larger-than-normal brain size or brain cell number to outstanding intellectual brilliance. And it by no means follows that there may be analogous situations for human singleton pregnancies, even though indi-

viduals in multiple human pregnancies would probably benefit
from having the other twin removed. They would only benefit
from reducing the mismatch between their achievement and their
potential.

Nutrition and Nutritionists

A very large part of the physiology and pathology of nutrition is
concerned with dietary composition rather than quantity of input
and with the characteristic effects of specific dietary deficiencies
whether "trace" substances or the more major dietary components
such as protein. Indeed the only mention of our subject in the
larger textbooks of clinical neurology is usually to be found in a
small chapter near the end on the neurological aspects of beri-beri
or Wernicke's encephalopathy or some other vitamin-deficiency
state. None of this is related to our present topic, in which there
are no longer any significant references to histopathological,
cerebral, or cellular lesions in the experimental literature, even
though certain descriptions of dog and pig neuropathology are
still endlessly quoted. As has been said before, the underprivileged countries are not widely populated by people with this
kind of neuropathology.

I certainly would not wish to enter the arena of the vexed international controversy known as the "protein fiasco." The protein-
lack mythology has played a great part in our own thinking, and
most experimental animal diets have been primarily protein deficient in intention. However, I have never been able to discover
any satisfactory evidence that protein deficiency has any specific
effect on the developing brain, in spite of the assumption on all
sides that it may have. Indeed it may be that for the developing
brain, just as some would say for most developing children, the
shortage is not of protein but of food.

This proposal is reinforced by yet another theoretical model
which tries to explain the known effects of undernutrition on the
developing physical brain, a pathology described as one of deficits and distortions[9] rather than of lesions. The organs and tissues of a child are not growing uniformly like a crystal grows, as
R. A. McCance would say. They grow asynchronously, and this
explains in part why the effects of growth restriction at different
stages are quite different in different tissues, and this leads to
quite different distortions of bodily relationships. You do not

merely miniaturize the growing child by undernutrition; you *distort* it. We know that the different regions of the brain grow in a similarly heterogeneous way.

It is to be expected, therefore, that growth restriction alone will similarly distort the gross and microscopical architecture of the brain in the way we do know actually happens. The best example is the greater effect on gross and microscopic structure of the cerebellum when the undernutrition is related to certain phases of cerebellar growth. This result can have nothing whatever to do with the quality of the diet. It would theoretically result from mere brain growth restriction, however caused. As I understand it, the "protein fiasco," according to those who believe it, really has been a fiasco, and has led to the application of important and expensive policies throughout the world which were wrongly conceived.

When applied to the brain, a similar series of mistakes could well be made, and so the matter is of considerable practical and political importance. Is it possible that the clearly different psychological temperaments of classical kwashiorkor and marasmus have misled people into proposing a specific effect of protein lack on the developing brain? The concurrent psychology of the malnourished child need have nothing to do with his residual problems following rehabilitation. There is certainly scope for confusion here, and we may have been confused. There was a time when fish was said to be good for the growing brain. Current attempts to relate precise dietary components to brain development center largely on the proposition in some quarters that the type of fatty acids in the diet can influence brain structural composition and ultimately behavioral factors. I know of no satisfactory evidence for this, and there is good circumstantial evidence from Svennerholm's laboratory to the contrary.

Biochemists in particular have shown great naïveté in this matter. Again the main practical importance of these things is the predictable manner in which important world health policy makers can be misled into supposing that dietary lactose, cystine, cholesterol, and polyenoic fatty acids go straight to the brain through some sort of tube connecting the mouth with nervous tissue and are there incorporated, molecule for molecule.[10] In fact, the brain shows an astonishing capacity for regulating its own intake of building blocks from the bloodstream during its development.

Indices of Structural Growth

The point has been made many times that we must not necessarily attribute tremendous functional and behavioral significance to those component substances in the brain which happen to be easy to estimate. Nevertheless, there are still those who endow brain DNA, or cholesterol, with almost mystical significance. Apart altogether from the limitations of DNA as an index of cell number in a tissue with such a heterogeneous cell population, the lay reader might be forgiven for understanding that DNA is the seat of the soul itself. Neither must we be swayed by this apparent denunciation of DNA and other commonly measured substances into believing that the useful days of DNA or cholesterol or water estimation are over. They probably have an unlimited life of usefulness still to come, provided they are used as *indices* of growth and not taken literally as representing the intellect. As said before, we have no notion of what, if anything, should be measured in the test tube to represent behavior, or intellect. If there should ever be such substances, they will almost certainly be difficult or impossible to measure; and the easily measured components may still lead us reliably to a detection of deficits and distortions in the things that matter. Thus, in a very narrow example, cholesterol is a much poorer index of myelin than the more specific myelin lipids. It remains an excellent index of myelination due to the apparently constant temporal and quantitative relationship between itself and the others, and it is infinitely easier to estimate in a few hundred samples.

Neurophysiology

Neurophysiology is a misnomer. It is a term mostly used to mean *electrophysiology*. My personal career began in neurophysiology. Perhaps because I was so bad at it, I quickly left the area with distinct prejudices about its very real but very limited usefulness. I do not think it is useful for horoscopes or for the detection of criminality; nor, I am afraid, do I see any part of it in our present subject.

Undernourished Human Brains

It is no criticism of anyone to say that the available information on human undernourished brains is almost worthless. Not only is

John Dobbing

this information subject to all the inevitable restrictions attributable to our methods of measuring them; it is also of hopelessly small number, and hopelessly undocumented. In most cases even fetal or postnatal age is not accurately known, and little trouble has been taken to relate the "brain anthropometry" to that of the rest of the child. Such elementary matters as the appropriateness or otherwise of a small brain for a small body can therefore rarely be discussed. The main reason for this mess is the extreme difficulty of properly collecting the human data and material. Some of the reason, however, is an apparent unwillingness to try. Most of the last year has been spent by one section of my own department on the regional analysis of more than 100 complete human brains taken from fetuses and newborn babies of mothers living in one of the most unfortunate and most indigent communities in the world. The main single difficulty in this kind of study is not having any satisfactory menstrual history from an illiterate and non-numerate population of mothers. There is, alas, no shortage of undernourished babies' brains. There is, however, a great shortage of those whose fetal age is accurately known. With the help of many collaborators we were able to identify a society whose cultural and religious practices insisted on an absolute recall of menstruation, and we therefore believe we shall shortly be able to answer at least the question whether human maternal malnutrition affects human fetal brain growth. At present it is too early to answer this question, but we already know that the incidence of low birth weight for gestational age is high, and there is an apparently corresponding reduction in brain dimensions and constituents. As set out elsewhere, however, these brains, had they lived, would almost certainly have been capable of good recovery. Such optimism stems from a reasonable extrapolation from animal models in which similar degrees of brain growth restriction were imposed for a similarly small, early proportion of their brain growth spurt, and which showed apparently full recovery following prompt rehabilitation. The optimism should, of course, be tempered by the realization that such children are rarely born into an environment where conditions conducive to rehabilitation actually occur.

Human Epidemiological Studies

The best (however incomplete) evidence that severe human maternal undernutrition during pregnancy does *not* deleteriously

affect the ultimate intellectual achievement of her offspring, provided there is reasonably prompt postnatal rehabilitation, comes
from the recent distinguished study by Stein et al.[11] of the wartime Dutch famine. It should be clearly understood, however, that
this whole study answers only the sharply circumscribed question, "Does acute, maternal undernutrition in humans, confined
to the pregnancy period, affect measured performance at 19 postnatal years in the male progeny?" The authors themselves emphasize, albeit in the very last sentence in the book, that their
findings "do not exclude prenatal nutrition as a possible factor *in
combination with poor postnatal nutrition*, especially in preindustrial societies" (my italics).

I wish this caveat could have been emblazoned as a running
headline on every page, since it is inevitable that important
people will be quite mistakenly reassured by such an excellent
study into a false belief that developmental malnutrition has no
detectable effect on human intellectual achievement at all.

The Stein et al. study must also be seen historically in relation
to our subject. It must have been designed in the years, not so long
ago, when it was believed that fetal life was the most vulnerable
period for human brain development; or at least that vulnerability
ended very soon after birth. Now that we believe that the human
brain growth spurt is predominantly postnatal and of much longer
duration than was formerly thought, the Stein et al. findings need
come as no great surprise, even if we assume a confined simplistic
relationship between undernutrition, brain "damage" and mental
retardation.

The Dutch famine was a remarkable "natural experiment." For
6 to 9 months large urban populations were fairly suddenly deprived of food, and even more suddenly relieved. Thus it is possible to consider quite sharply circumscribed cohorts of individuals
according to the stage of their fetal and postnatal life when they
were severely undernourished. Now, assuming that the main effect of maternal starvation on human fetal growth begins at about
30 weeks of gestation (and the authors confirmed this), the most
seriously affected individuals would probably be the cohort who
entered their third trimester at the beginning of the famine and
were liberated from it when they were 6 postnatal months old.
When it is remembered that these babies must have been breastfed (which promotes good baby growth even in malnourished
mothers), and that their last fetal trimester imposed only relatively

minor growth restriction because of the expected relative sparing of the fetus, it will be seen that brain growth could not be expected to have been very much impaired even in the worst affected cohorts. Since the human brain growth spurt lasts at least until the second birthday, and probably beyond, and since this was a sophisticated western society that would immediately "rehabilitate" its mothers and children well within the vulnerable period on the reappearance of supplies, it is reasonable to conclude (again from properly extrapolated animal models) that no measurable harm to the physical brain would have resulted.

All this, however, assumes that nutrition and growth rate are the only important factors. If we return to the algebraic sum hypothesis mentioned at the beginning, a number of other important special features can be discerned. There was a sharp decline in the number of conceptions which survived. Are we then left with a selected population, selected for their biological fitness? The Dutch people are not uneducated. They had long had a rationing plan for the eventuality of food shortage which gave some priority to such groups as pregnant mothers and children, and as individuals they may well have augmented the differential still further. Fathers may well have preferentially starved themselves in favor of their babies and their pregnant wives. Such facts as these cannot emerge from retrospective epidemiological surveys of average food distribution. When we consider the non-nutritional factors in the algebraic sum, is it not likely that the mother-child interactional contribution would in these desperate emergency circumstances have been heavily augmented in favor of the baby? And what reliance can we place on Dutch military IQ's as a measure of the reality of intellectual achievement we require for our present discussion?

For these, our present purposes, I much prefer the continuing studies of previously malnourished Jamaican children begun under the inspiration of Herbert Birch, with great insight into their inevitable limitations, a study being carried on now by Stephen Richardson. I think it is mistaken of Stein et al. to compare the Jamaica study with the negative results of J. D. Hansen in South Africa in order to contrast their findings. One of the many problems with human field investigation is that no one study can be properly compared with any other. They are too dissimilar in too many important ways.

Lastly, I hope I may be forgiven for assuming a sufficient acquaintance with the subject to make detailed references super-fluous. I make no apology for expressing a purely personal point of view.

References

1. Cabak, V., and R. Najdanvic. Effect of undernutrition in early life on physical and mental development. *Arch. Dis. Child.* 40: 532, 1965.
2. Cravioto, J., and B. Robles. Evolution of adaptive and motor behavior during rehabilitation from kwashiorkor. *Am. J. Orthopsychiat.* 35: 449, 1965.
3. Dobbing, J. The influence of early nutrition on the development and myelination of the brain. *Proc. Roy. Soc. Biol.* 159: 503, 1964.
4. Dobbing, J. Effects of experimental undernutrition on development of the nervous system. In *Malnutrition, Learning and Behavior*, N. S. Scrimshaw and J. E. Gordon, eds., M.I.T. Press, Cambridge, Mass., 1968.
5. Dobbing, J. Vulnerable period in developing brain. In *Applied Neurochemistry*, A. N. Davison and J. Dobbing, eds., Blackwell Scientific Pub. Ltd., Oxford, 1968.
6. Dobbing, J. In *Scientific Foundations of Paediatrics*, J. A. Davis and J. Dobbing, eds., Heinemann, London, and Saunders, Philadelphia, 1974.
7. Dobbing, J., and J. Smart. Vulnerability of developing brain and behavior. *Brit. Med. Bull.* 30: 164, 1974.
8. Dobbing, J., and E. M. Widdowson. The effect of undernutrition and subsequent rehabilitation on myelination of rat brain as measured by its composition. *Brain* 88: 357, 1965.
9. Jelliffe, D. B., and E. F. P. Jelliffe. Human milk, nutrition, and the world resource crisis. *Science* 188: 557, 1975.
10. Platt, B. S., R. J. C. Stewart, and S. M. Payne. Protein-calorie deficiency and the nervous system. In *Variation in Chemicals of the Central Nervous System as Determined by Developmental and Genetic Factors*, G. B. Ansell, ed., Oxford, London, and Pergamon Press, New York, 1966.
11. Stein, Z., M. Susser, G. Saenger, and F. Marolla. *Famine and Human Development*, Oxford University Press, New York, 1975.
12. Stoch, M. B., and P. M. Smythe. Does undernutrition during infancy inhibit brain growth and subsequent intellectual development? *Arch. Dis. Child.* 38: 548, 1963.
13. Widdowson, E. M., and R. A. McCance. The effect of finite periods of undernutrition at different ages on the composition and subsequent development of the rat. *Proc. Roy. Soc. Biol.* 158: 329, 1960.
14. Winick, M., and A. Noble. Cellular response in rats during malnutrition at various ages. *J. Nutr.* 89: 300, 1966.

Stephen Zamenhof and Edith van Marthens 5

Study of Some Nutritional and Regulatory Factors Affecting Prenatal Brain Development

Introduction

At the root of our present ideas on the effects of malnutrition on behavioral development are three independent concepts. One is that brain development is not a completely gene-predetermined, unchangeable entity, but that development can be modified by the environment; to use Myron Winick's expression, brain development can be *manipulated*, in plus or in minus. Another concept is that nutrition is an important tool or factor for this brain manipulation. A third concept, of particular interest to us, is that since so much of the brain development takes place before birth, considerable manipulation of this development should be possible even prenatally.

In the past, all three concepts were confronted with the prejudices of their times. Right after the early triumphs of genetics it was inconceivable that such an important organ as the brain could be influenced by something as unpredictable as the environment. Unlike liver or muscle tissue, brain was "spared" in many cases of malnutrition, so it was "safe." And the fetus was a "parasite," extracting from the mother all it needed, thus being immune to prenatal (maternal) malnutrition.

In spite of these assumptions, the author embarked on a project in 1940–1942 aimed at increasing the number of brain neurons by early treatment with pituitary growth hormone. The 1941 work on tadpoles[57] was recently confirmed,[32] indicating that early brain development can be stimulated. Conclusions by ourselves[47, 58] and others[15] on the effect of growth hormone injection into pregnant rats, however, were too premature. As we found out later,[71] the positive results might have been due not to growth hormone *per se*, but to prenatal nutrition (mobilization of maternal nutrient reserves). We will return to this subject later.

After studying factors that *stimulated* prenatal brain development, it was natural that we look for those that might depress it. The most obvious of these seemed malnutrition. This was not our own idea. When we were able to resume this work in 1966, thanks to the liberal research atmosphere at the University of California at Los Angeles (UCLA), studies of the effects of malnutrition on *postnatal* brain development were already under way.

In 1966 Richard Barnes and his collaborators published the fundamental paper[5] on the influence of nutritional deprivations in early life on learning behavior of rats as measured by performance in a water maze. In his work on rats, the nutritional deprivations were imposed in three ways. First, rats were foster-nursed from the second to the twenty-first day of life in large litters of 14 or 16 per lactating female. Second, rats were fed a low-protein diet (3 to 4 percent) for 8 weeks from weaning, and third, rats were double-deprived by nursing in large litters and then weaning to the low-protein diet. Five to 9 months after rehabilitation from these three forms of malnutrition the rats were studied in a discrimination test involving a Y-shaped water maze. After 50 trials, 2 each day, all rats had reached a criterion of 20 percent or less errors. There was, however, a repeatable and significant difference in the rate of learning, favoring the control rats (8 per litter and fed a normal diet after weaning) over the double-deprived rats. In his later work, varying degrees of malnutrition were imposed on pigs from the third through the eleventh week of life. [4,6] The general conclusion[7] was that restricting the intake of a food of normal composition in early life may have had longlasting effects upon certain behavioral characteristics.

Encouraged by these results, we began to look for other evidence. There were the animal studies of Cowley and Griesel,[16-18] and Caldwell and Churchill,[11] all on behavioral aspects of early malnutrition. There were papers by Chow and his collaborators[12,31] on the general effects of early malnutrition on body weights and growth of the young. Dobbing, Widdowson and their collaborators studied the "growth spurts" in animal brains and developed the important concept of "vulnerable periods" in developing brains.[19-21, 25] Winick and Noble studied the increases in brain DNA content during development[53] and pointed out the importance of discerning between reduction in glial cell number and reduction in glial cell size during postnatal malnutrition; this led to recognition of irreversible and reversible damages.[54] Zeman[76] studied the effects of maternal protein restriction on the young rat.

This short historical note cannot mention all the workers in the field, nor can it give justice to all work done by the mentioned authors; it was meant only to emphasize that at that time the climate was ripe for our work. As mentioned previously, we were committed to prenatal effects.

Fetal Malnutrition

As it is recognized now, fetal malnutrition (including embryonal malnutrition) can have at least two components: (1) maternal malnutrition during pregnancy, and/or (2) placental insufficiency. These components are interdependent, and our work on both of them will be discussed together. In 1968, with Margolis, we demonstrated[75] that when female rats were maintained on an 8 or 27 percent casein diet for 1 month before mating and throughout gestation, the brains of newborn rats from females on the 8 percent casein diet contained significantly less DNA and protein compared to the progeny of the females on the 27 percent casein diet. The data on DNA indicated there were fewer cells;[60, 62] the protein content per cell was also lower. If, at birth, the brain cells are predominantly neurons, and their number becomes final at that time,[66, 68] then such dietary restriction may result in some permanent brain neuron deficiency. This alteration in cell number as well as protein content per cell may constitute a basis for the impaired behavior of the offspring from protein-deprived mothers.

Around that time Winick[50] and Zeman[77] worked independently on similar problems so that our results were soon confirmed.

Our findings indicated that malnutrition during pregnancy alone was much less harmful than malnutrition started one month before mating and continued through pregnancy. Thus, there was evidence that maternal nutrient reserves at the beginning of pregnancy were an important factor in determining the outcome of malnourished pregnancy.

Intrigued by the problem of *timing* of prenatal malnutrition, we decided to divide the pregnancy itself into shorter periods of malnutrition. In order to get demonstrable effects, the dietary restriction of the mother had to be more rigorous: a protein-free diet. Pregnant rats were fed a protein-free diet during five periods of pregnancy: days 0 to 10, 10 to 15, 13 to 18, 15 to 20, or 10 to 20. During the remaining time until parturition they were given an adequate protein diet.[69] In 62 percent of the dams fed a protein-free diet from days 0 to 10, there was a failure to litter. There was no significant change in the food intake in any of the groups; yet in all cases there were significant decreases in body weights, cerebral weights, cerebral DNA, and cerebral protein of their offspring, even though until day 15, the total protein increment of the embryo and its supporting tissue constitutes only an insignificant fraction (1.3 percent) of the average maternal protein intake. Thus, the observed effects were unlikely to be due to an actual deficiency of amino acids per se as required for embryonal protein synthesis. Work in other laboratories demonstrated that the effects described above could be traced to deficient placental development caused by a deficiency in estrogen and progesterone, caused, in turn, by a deficiency in maternal pituitary gonadotropic hormones. The latter might presumably be triggered by a change in amino acid balance (or serum proteins) acting in the pituitary and/or the hypothalamus that produces pituitary hormone-releasing factors. After day 11, when the placenta starts to assume the hormonal functions of the maternal pituitary, the deficiency in placental development may further contribute to the overall effect. Winick[51] reported adverse effects of maternal protein restriction on placental development as early as day 13. Our data on the 16- and 20-day Caesarean following deprivation from days 10 to 15 also indicated deficient placental development. This deficiency persisted to term (20-day Caesarean).

After day 15, the total protein increments of the fetus and its supporting tissue cease to be insignificant. Brain underdevelopment due to protein deprivation after this time may be due to a direct deficiency of amino acids required for protein synthesis. The adverse effect on the development of the placenta may also continue. The most pronounced effects were obtained by protein deprivation from days 10 to 20. This seems to indicate the cumulative effect of both these mechanisms.

Thus, at least in the rat, pregnancy operates on a very tight schedule. There is no second chance; a growth phase missed or slowed down by malnutrition even for a short time cannot be rehabilitated by subsequent normal feeding. The mechanisms involved are complex. It is of interest that one of these mechanisms (resorption of fetuses) has been developed during evolution to protect the mother against the organisms of different genomes (fetuses). Evidently in times of emergency (protein deprivation) it is better to preserve a normal mother than to produce subnormal offspring. Obviously the evolutionary driving force here was the selection for the features fittest to the species as a whole, rather than the selection of the fittest individual genomes (fetus versus fetus or fetus versus mother).

It has been found that in the human, neuron proliferation terminates early.[23, 24] This has been recently interpreted[22, 24] as meaning that in the human, proliferation of brain neurons cannot be affected by prenatal malnutrition because, that early in pregnancy, the nutrient requirements of the fetus are still negligible ("highly protected second trimester"). We disagree with this interpretation. We do not feel that even the earliest pregnancy is highly protected. As discussed above, there is evidence[69] that rat embryos are usually destroyed (resorbed) a few days after implantation if the maternal diet lacks protein. This occurs even though at that stage the rat embryo requires (comparatively) even less protein than the human fetus in the second trimester. The embryos that do survive exhibit deficient placenta and brain development. A strict regulatory mechanism is in control rather than the amount of food required by the embryo at that time.

In the course of the above experiments we obtained evidence that the normally nourished female offspring (F_1) of mothers (F_0) malnourished during pregnancy will produce offspring (F_2) that still have significantly lower brain parameters.[72, 73] This transfer of deficiencies to the F_2 generation is only through F_1 females, not through F_1 males; it is not a Mendelian inheritance. Several possible explanations have to be considered. Poor lactation of F_0 nursing mothers was not the cause. The effects on the brain in F_2 in another group were essentially the same, although the nursing mothers were never protein-restricted.

Possible explanations of the effect on the brain in F_2 animals may include the following. Due to protein restriction of F_0 mothers before delivery, the F_1 offspring are born handicapped, not only with regard to the brain[75] but also in other respects. Hall and Zeman[29] have reported that the offspring of rats similarly protein-restricted during pregnancy suffer from retardation of kidney development and altered kidney function. Lee and Chow[33] have reported that the restricted progeny showed reduced feed efficiency and low nitrogen balance; they excreted more amino acids than the controls. Thus, each progeny (F_1) may have suffered from cryptic malnutrition, even when postnatally given full access to normal food, and, as a result, their progeny (F_2) had a cerebral cell deficiency.[75]

Another possibility is that the F_1 organs affected were endocrine glands. Stephan et al.[41] have recently shown that similar F_1 animals had smaller pituitaries containing lower concentrations of growth hormone. Deficiencies of this and possibly other maternal (F_1) hormones may have affected fetal brain development of the F_2 offspring.

Other cases of maternal inheritance are well known, but the implications of the preceding case may be of particular interest. They reveal the existence of a long-range regulatory mechanism which, generation after generation, cumulatively adjusts the size of individuals and their organs (within genetic limits) to the nutritional opportunities confronting a given strain. Thus, what we consider a deficiency may actually mean an adjustment that has a selective value for survival of the species. A recent study of birth weights[39] indicates that such phenomena may be operating also in humans. The degree of constraint imposed on the fetus is correlated with the degree of constraint experienced by the mother when she herself was a fetus.

Encouraged by Barnes's work with the water maze[5] as well as his later work with Levitsky[34,35] and Fraňková,[26,27] we arranged collaboration with Bressler and Ellison of our psychology department[10] to test the learning ability of the F_2 offspring in a water maze; this learning ability was found to be significantly impaired.[59] The study was then repeated in a specially designed computerized maze[10] with essentially similar results. Thus, Cowley's results,[18] published in 1966, were essentially confirmed.

In all the above experiments the maternal dietary restriction was in protein as such. However, what reaches the fetus is not the intact protein but the amino acids. Thus, the next step was to investigate the effect of exclusion of single amino acids, especially essential amino acids, from the maternal diet.

A protein-free diet containing a complete chemically defined mixture of L-amino acids (AA) or this mixture deprived of one of the essential amino acids (tryptophan, lysine, or methionine) was fed to pregnant rats.[64] The feeding period was 0 to 21 or 10 to 21

61

days of pregnancy. At birth the following newborn parameters were measured: body weight, cerebral weight, cerebral DNA (cell number), and cerebral protein, as well as placental weight, placental DNA, and placental protein. Compared with a normal (pelleted) stock diet, the AA diet resulted in small decreases that were significant for body weight and cerebral parameters, though not significant for placental parameters; thus it still remains uncertain whether our present knowledge of nutritional factors for optimal fetal development is sufficient to devise a faultless synthetic diet for pregnancy. The need for "unknown growth factors" cannot yet be excluded.

Omission of tryptophan, lysine, or methionine from the AA diet resulted in offspring significantly inferior to the AA diet offspring in all parameters. The deficiencies were essentially similar to those produced in our previous study by total protein deprivation.[69,75] Thus, omission of single essential amino acids during pregnancy may be as harmful as total absence of dietary protein. Such a study may be of importance in view of the well-known single or double essential amino acid deficiencies in many foods of plant origin.

In all the above experiments the maternal dietary restriction was in protein only, while caloric intake was kept normal. However, since glucose is the main energy source for the fetus, it was of interest to see whether restriction of caloric intake alone (with normal protein intake) would also affect prenatal brain development. We found[70,71] that such restriction of caloric intake to one-third of normal, even during the second half of pregnancy only, resulted in highly significant decreases in neonatal body weight, placental weight, neonatal cerebral weight, cerebral DNA (cell number), and cerebral protein. It was gratifying for us to hear from Habicht and his collaborators[28] about his evidence of the importance of caloric supplementation in prevention of incidence of "small for date" babies.

In the past we have been impressed by the work of Altman[2] and other anatomists who were trying to demonstrate the postnatal damage to the developing brain caused by many factors.

In close collaboration with L. Kruger of our department of anatomy an attempt was made to visualize the effects of prenatal caloric malnutrition on neonatal and older brains. Cerebral cell number, although intimately involved in brain performance,[30,46] is not directly related to other factors of brain function such as the extent of the neuronal dendritic tree.[15,46] Cortical thickness and cortical cross-sectional area, on the other hand, should reflect both the cell number and the development of cellular arborization. We were concerned therefore with the problem whether cortical thickness and area are also reduced by prenatal caloric restriction.[14] The restriction was imposed from day 10 to day 20 of pregnancy. The experimental diet contained 1.39 Kcal/g compared to 3.330 Kcal/g in the control diet. At birth, at 10 days of age, and at adulthood, the brains were dissected out; on some, cerebral DNA (cell number) and cerebral protein were determined as described above. Other brains, to be studied histologically, were placed immediately in formalin and fixed for a minimum of 10 days. Serial 50 μm frozen coronal sections were cut, mounted, and stained with cresyl-violet for quantitative study. Stained sections at the rostral and caudal poles of the corpus callosum were selected and their projections traced for subsequent measurements.

We found that not only cerebral parameters of the offspring (weight, DNA, protein) but also cortical dimensions (thickness at several positions, width, area) were significantly reduced when pregnant rats were maintained on calorie-deficient diets. The reduction in cortical thickness was approximately double that expected from the reduction in cerebral weight, which suggests that the cortex itself is more affected by such malnutrition than the cerebrum as a whole. We also found that all these decreases were more pronounced at birth than at 10 days or in later development. Thus, for visualization of prenatal deficiencies one should study the brain at birth or shortly thereafter. Although it is more difficult to demonstrate the deficiencies later on, this does not mean rehabilitation after birth has occurred, because by then the neurons have practically ceased to proliferate; it means that after birth the damages become hidden due to differentiation and considerable brain expansion.

All the above work was concerned with one component of fetal malnutrition, namely maternal malnutrition during pregnancy. In 1964, Wigglesworth[48] laid the foundations for experimental study of the second component of fetal malnutrition, namely the deficiency of placental transfer. He has produced experimental uteroplacental ischemia in rat pups by occluding the uterine artery for varying time periods. Such ischemia produced a varying degree of stunting. The individual organs were differentially affected, depending on their growth rate after the time of vascular occlusion. The brain itself was less affected than the body as a whole. Similar results were obtained by Winick.[52] In his experiments the total cell number in the brain was not affected.

We thought that it would be of interest to find an animal model in which ischemia produces demonstrable brain underdevelopment, as it seems to occur in "small for date" human infants. For these experiments we chose the rabbit, which in many respects is a better model for human perinatal brain development. Experimental ischemia was induced during the last trimester by ligation of spiral arterioles, and the differential effects on fetal development at term were demonstrated.[44] Specific brain regions were examined for wet weight, total cell number (DNA), and total protein content. Highly significant decreases in all these parameters were found in both the cortex and cerebellum following the above-mentioned experimental intrauterine growth retardation; these two organs were differentially affected.

In summary, fetal malnutrition and fetal brain underdevelopment cover a multitude of sins. This should be obvious if one considers the multitude of potential *regulatory* sites on which fetal neuronal proliferation depends. Figure 5.1 represents a simplified schematic diagram of the flow of nutrients to the site of synthesis of neuronal (neuroblast) components of the embryo or fetus.[67] Maternal dietary nutrients themselves (Figure 5.1, upper bracket) are only part of the story.

Maternal dietary nutrients, digested, absorbed, and ultimately available in the blood, can be supplemented by substances (such as nonessential amino acids) manufactured in maternal organs, primarily liver, and by vitamins manufactured by the intestinal flora. The amounts of nutrients may be further decreased or increased by the participation of maternal nutrient reserves. In particular, one of the hormones mobilizing these reserves is the pituitary growth hormone. The blood level of this hormone is known to increase during fasting and during pregnancy. We have demonstrated[71] that growth hormone administered to the nutritionally deprived mother prevents the deficiencies in cerebral DNA and protein in the offspring (see further).

It is now well recognized that the fetus is not a parasite that extracts from the maternal organism all it needs; rather, the fetus may be sacrificed to save the mother. This is particularly well demonstrated in the rat. As mentioned above, maternal dietary

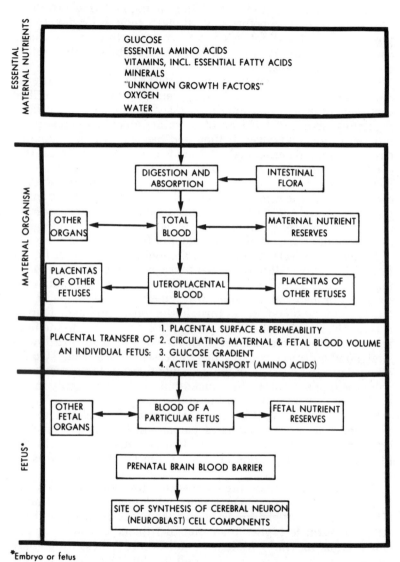

*Embryo or fetus

Figure 5.1. Scheme of flow of nutrients to the fetus and the role of nutrient reserves

protein deprivation around the time of implantation results in resorption of fetuses before day 10, even though by day 15 the protein content of all fetuses and their supporting tissues would constitute only an insignificant fraction of the total protein intake of the pregnant female.[69]

Proper placental transfer of nutrients to the fetus is a key requirement for normal fetal development. In the above-described case, lack of proper placentation, caused by the consequences of regulatory action of the lack of proteins, precluded subsequent transfer of nutrients even if they had become available. As discussed earlier, maternal malnutrition is one of the conditions that causes placental underdevelopment. Thus, lack of nutrients may have a twofold effect: deficiency of transfer to the fetus and deficiency of substances to be transferred. This deficiency of transfer due to placental underdevelopment might also affect the passage of "nutrients" present in abundance, such as oxygen and water, as well as the removal of waste material from the fetus.

As mentioned earlier, glucose is the main energy source for the fetus. The factor determining the passage of glucose through the placenta appears to be the concentration gradient (although the carrier is probably also involved). Glucose concentrations in maternal and fetal blood are, in turn, hormonally regulated. Thus, it is possible, for example, to increase glucose transport to the fetus by introducing more insulin to the fetus, which in turn lowers fetal blood glucose level and thus increases the gradient.[40] On the other hand, the passage of amino acids through the placenta involves active transport: the concentration of amino acids in the fetal blood is higher than in the maternal.[9]

From the foregoing it is clear that placental development and placental transfer are factors of paramount importance for fetal brain development; but the problem of quantification in the placenta is a difficult one because of the number of factors involved.

Then, there is intrauterine competition (in most mammals and in multiple births of humans). It is well known that in humans, birth weight of singletons is higher than that of twins, and the latter, in turn, is higher than that of triplets and quadruplets. However, as shown by McKeown and Record[36] these differences appear only after 26 weeks of gestation. Until that time there are enough nutrients and even enough space for each of quadruplets to be the same size as singletons.

Recently Dobbing and Sands demonstrated that in human brains the termination of neuron proliferation may occur on the twentieth week of pregnancy[23] or even earlier[24] (except for short-axon neurons in some parts of the brain.[1] Thus, during evolution an efficient regulatory mechanism has been developed to prevent restriction of size in multiple births during the period in which neurons still proliferate. This should result in the same number of neurons in multiple as in single births, but in humans this subject has not been investigated. Nevertheless, although the neuron proliferation in the human may be exempt from competition, glial (glioblast) proliferation, which occurs later,[23,24] may depend on the number in the litter, even at full maternal nutrition. The following study may or may not be related to this situation. Twenty sets of twins of the same sex with weight differences of 300 g or more at birth and a gestation period of at least 36 weeks were examined for intellectual achievement at the mean age of 8.5 years. The results showed that the twin underweight at birth exhibited a significantly lower level of intellectual achievement in the areas examined.[3]

Correlations

Correlations between parameters of normal population are (sometimes) useful for establishing *functional* relationships. To give an historical example, the harmful effects of smoking during pregnancy were discovered mainly on the basis of statistical correlations.

The results of Winick's[51] and our [69] studies of the effect of malnutrition on placental development encouraged us to attempt to correlate placental size with newborn brain parameters. As mentioned above, the problem of quantification in the placental function is a difficult one because of the number of factors involved. The permeability of the placenta, the exchange surface, the maternal blood flow to the placenta, and the placental enzyme and hormone production are all involved. Of these, blood flow to the uterus appears to increase in proportion to the placental weight,[8] and therefore the weight was chosen as a placental parameter to study.[61] Our work was done on eighty rabbit fetuses and their placentas, removed at term. We found that on a statistical basis, an individual animal with a heavier term placenta is also likely to have higher neonatal cerebral weight. The latter is also likely to have a higher number of neonatal cerebral cells (DNA).

Thus, the factors that limit the development of one fetal organ (placenta) indirectly also limit the development of other organs, for example, the brain. It has been suggested[37] that the retardation of growth of the fetus toward term is due, not to the inability of the fetus to maintain its rate of growth, but to the inability of the prenatal environment to fully meet the needs of the fetus.

In humans the data on neonatal brain weight and neonatal cerebral cell number (DNA) are rarely available. For this reason our study in humans had to be limited to the study of correlations between placental parameters on one side, and neonatal weight and neonatal head circumference on the other side. Earlier studies by Winick and Rosso[56] indicated that there is a linear relation between head circumference and brain DNA (cell number) during the first year of life of essentially normal human infants. Our study[65] was made on 55 male and 36 female normal infants born at the UCLA Hospital. We found that placental weight, placental DNA (cell number), and placental protein were all well correlated with each other. We also found that on a statistical basis, an infant with a heavier placenta is also likely to have a larger neonatal head circumference and, therefore, presumably more brain DNA (cell number).

The demonstration of the statistically significant correlations between brain parameters and neonatal body weight also appears to be of importance; and, in humans and other animals studied, neonatal body weight is significantly correlated with placental weight,[61, 65] (see also reviews[38, 74]), and, as discussed above, correlated with the nutritional status of the mother.[51, 73, 75] Since body weight is often the only parameter that is routinely available at birth, the foresaid correlations, if established, will make it possible to estimate, on the basis of neonatal body weights, the concomitant neonatal brain development. The estimate would be statistically valid for a population, though it may not be valid in individual cases. For this reason, we made an attempt to establish such correlations in a large rat population: 249 neonatal (29 litters) and 107 adult normal rats.[63] It was found that, on a statistical basis, an individual with a heavier neonatal body weight is also likely to have a higher cerebral weight, neonatal cerebral DNA (cell number), and neonatal cerebral protein. For a sample of this size, each pair of these parameters was significantly correlated. In adult animals the significance of correlations with body weights disappears, but the correlations between each pair of cerebral parameters remain significant.

Thus, statistically, one can predict brain parameters from body weights, but only in neonatal animals. In the mature animals, these correlations were obscured by the general body and brain growth.

We found a similar situation when we studied correlations between cerebral and *cortical* parameters.[13] Body and brain parameters were measured in newborns and in 10-day-old and mature rats. In the rostral sections of the newborn brains, cortical areas, cortical thickness in all positions measured, and cerebral widths were significantly correlated with each other. Cortical thicknesses were also well correlated with cerebral weights. In 10-day-old rats, the rostral and some caudal sections show significant correlation between each pair of the cortical thicknesses, and between cortical thicknesses and cerebral widths. At this age, body weight is also correlated with cerebral weight and with almost every one of the rostral and caudal cortical thicknesses, as well as with the caudal cerebral width. In the mature animal all these correlations tend to become obscured by the body and brain growth. In general, the measurement of only one brain parameter at a specific age does not allow one to draw conclusions about the overall development of the cortex; however, any such measurements are better correlated at birth or at 10 days than in the mature brain.

Supernutrition

At present it is difficult to ascertain whether a particular dietary regime that does not give any symptoms of malnutrition is also an *optimal* regime. Differences in strains, intestinal absorption, and so on may play a considerable role. A diet optimal in one respect or at one time in development may not be so in other respects or at other times. We are, here, mainly concerned with the conditions *optimal for prenatal brain development.*

The term "supernutrition" as distinct from "overnutrition" has been used by Williams[49] to denote "quality above and beyond nutrition as it is ordinarily experienced" to provide "a completely suitable assortment ideally tailored to individual needs." While this concept as presented here has mainly qualitative connotations, the optimal *quantity* is also a part of supernutrition. In 1967 Winick and Noble[55] reported that increasing the quantity of milk available to rat pups during nursing resulted in an increase in cell number of many organs, including the brain.

We found, however, that the quantity of nutrients, normally assigned by the mother to a fetus, may not be optimal and is subject to experimental improvement.

One part of our work is a continuation of our study on the effects of pituitary growth hormone (see introduction). In the case of maternal malnutrition during pregnancy, which results in malnourished fetuses, one may wonder if the mother is supplying all the nutrients she can. After all, she usually has ample nutrient reserves: fat, glycogen, muscle protein, if only she were able to mobilize them.

The levels of pituitary growth hormone are known to increase during pregnancy and during fasting. Perhaps this is for the purpose of mobilizing maternal nutrient reserves or, at least, of preventing deposition of fat. Thus, mothers of similar genome but different pituitary development might produce offspring of different brain development. In maternal malnutrition such natural mobilization is often not sufficient to produce normal offspring.

We attempted to stimulate nutrient mobilization by injecting pregnant females with additional growth hormone.[71] We found that such treatment of malnourished females produced nearly normal offspring. The improvements of the malnourished animals were statistically highly significant. In addition, treatment of normally nourished females with growth hormone produced a significant increase in cerebral weight over and above the normal. This increase was not due to water but to increased content of cerebral protein. As explained above, the primary action of this hormone might have been on the mother, by mobilization of maternal nutrient reserves, especially fat deposits. Thus, conceivably, each fetus received more nutrients which stimulated its prenatal brain development.

Another way of enhancing neonatal brain development is to reduce operatively the number of fetuses during pregnancy. Presumably this procedure also provides more nutrients per surviving fetus. The result is a significant increase in neonatal body weight, placental weight, cerebral weight, cerebral DNA (cell number) and cerebral protein.[42,43,45] One method of achieving this reduction consists in tying one of the two uterine horns (in the rat) prior to mating.[45] Another method, which we used in rabbits[42] and rats,[43] consists in destroying some implantation sites soon

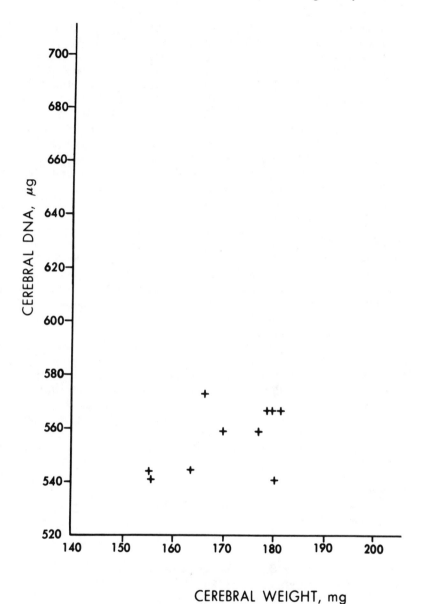

Figure 5.2 Cerebral DNA content as a function of cerebral weight

after implantation. In rabbits, the increases were up to 105 percent in placental weight, up to 50 percent in neonatal body weight, up to 21 percent in cerebral DNA (cell number), and up to 46 percent in cerebral protein. In the rat[43] the increases in placental weights closely followed the degree of reduction of number of fetuses.

The remarkable constancy of neonatal cerebral DNA (cell number)[66, 67, 74] in normal animals is probably the result of stringent regulatory mechanisms. Conceivably, they consist of a multitude of closely overlapping checks so that if one factor is enhanced, the next one becomes the rate-limiting step, and so on. Nevertheless, cases of enhanced brain development in genetically uniform strains not only can be produced experimentally but also occur naturally. In natural cases it is possible that many factors have changed in concert.

As can be seen from Figure 5.2, in a genetically uniform population animals can be found which have brain DNA well above the range of others (more than 2 std. dev.) from the same litter.[67] Such spontaneous occurrences are rare—in approximately 2 percent of the cases in the rat. The causes of such high DNA are completely unknown, but their occurrence indicates that the mechanisms of regulation of DNA synthesis and cell number in prenatal brain are not completely precise and inviolable.

It is tacitly implied that what we find in animals can, with some reservations, be applied also to humans. Thus, behavioral deficiencies due to brain underdevelopment in animals may correspond to mental retardation in humans. We hope that such studies will lead eventually to some degree of prevention in certain cases of mental retardation. But if the production of superior intellects, or intellects optimal within genetic limits, were ever possible, would it not have a far greater impact on our civilization than just prevention of mental retardation?

Acknowledgements

This research was supported by USPHS grants HD-05615 and HD-08927.

References

1. Altman, J., and G. D. Das. Autographic and histological studies of postnatal neurogenesis. I. A longitudinal investigation of the kinetics, migration and transformation of cells incorporating tritiated thymidine in neonate rats, with special reference to postnatal neurogenesis in some brain regions. *J. Comp. Neurol.* 126: 337, 1966.

2. Altman, J., and B. McCrady. The influence of nutrition on neural and behavioral development. IV. Effects of infantile undernutrition on the growth of the cerebellum. *Devel. Psychobiol.* 5: 111, 1972.
3. Babson, G. S., J. Kangas, N. Young, and J. L. Bramhall. Growth and development of twins of dissimilar size at birth. *Pediatrics* 33: 327, 1964.
4. Barnes, R. H. Experimental animal approaches to the study of early malnutrition and mental development. *Fed. Proc.* 26: 144, 1967.
5. Barnes, R. H., S. R. Cunnold, R. R. Zimmermann, H. Simmons, R. B. MacLeod, and L. Krook. Influence of nutritional deprivations in early life on learning behavior of rats as measured by performance in a water maze. *J. Nutr.* 89: 399, 1966.
6. Barnes, R. H., A. U. Moore, I. M. Reid, and W. G. Pond. Learning behavior following nutritional deprivations in early life. *J. Am. Dietet. Assn.* 51: 34, 1967.
7. Barnes, R. H., A. U. Moore, I. M. Reid, and W. G. Pond. Effect of food deprivation on behavioral patterns. In *Malnutrition, Learning, and Behavior*, N. S. Scrimshaw and J. E. Gordon, eds., M.I.T. Press, Cambridge, Mass., 1968, p. 203.
8. Barron, D. H. Homeostasis of the foetus. In *Congenital Malformations*, M. Fishbein, ed., Lippincott, Phila., 1960, p. 247.
9. Blaxter, K. L. Protein metabolism and requirements in pregnancy and lactation. In *Mammalian Protein Metabolism*, II, H. N. Munro and J. B. Allison, eds., Academic Press, New York, 1964.
10. Bressler, D., G. Ellison, and S. Zamenhof. Learning deficits in rats with malnourished grandmothers. *Devel. Psychobiol.* 8: 315, 1975.
11. Caldwell, D. F., and J. A. Churchill. Learning ability in the progeny of rats administered a protein-deficient diet during the second half of gestation. *Neurol.* 17: 95, 1967.
12. Chow, B. F., and C. J. Lee. Effect of dietary restriction of pregnant rats on body weight gain of the offspring. *J. Nutr.* 82: 10, 1964.
13. Clark, G. M., and S. Zamenhof. Correlations between cerebral and cortical parameters in the developing and mature rat brain. *Internat. J. Neurosci.* 5: 223, 1973.
14. Clark, G. M., S. Zamenhof, E. van Marthens, L. Grauel, and L. Kruger. The effects of prenatal malnutrition on dimensions of cerebral cortex. *Brain Res.* 54: 397, 1973.
15. Clendinnen, B. G., and J. T. Eayrs. The anatomical and physiological effects of prenatally administered somatotrophin on cerebral development in rats. *J. Endocri.* 22: 183, 1961.
16. Cowley, J. J., and R. D. Griesel. Some effects of a low protein diet on a first filial generation of white rats. *J. Genet. Psychol.* 95: 187, 1959.
17. Cowley, J. J., and R. D. Griesel. The development of second-generation low-protein rats. *J. Genet. Psychol.* 103: 233, 1963.
18. Cowley, J. J., and R. D. Griesel. The effect on growth and behavior of rehabilitating first and second generation low protein rats. *Anim. Behav.* 14: 506, 1966.

19. Davison, A. N., and J. Dobbing. Myelination as a vulnerable period in brain development. *Brit. Med. Bull.* 22: 40, 1966.
20. Dickerson, J. W. T., and J. Dobbing. Prenatal and postnatal growth and development of the central nervous system of the pig. *Proc. Roy. Soc. Biol.* 166: 384, 1967.
21. Dickerson, J. W. T., J. Dobbing, and R. A. McCance. The effect of undernutrition on the postnatal development of the brain and cord in pigs. *Proc. Roy. Soc. Biol.* 166: 396, 1967.
22. Dobbing, J. Prenatal nutrition and neurological development. In *Symp. Swedish Nutr. Found.*, XII, Almquist and Wiksell, Uppsala, 1974, p. 96.
23. Dobbing, J., and J. Sands. Timing of neuroblast multiplication in developing human brain. *Nature* (London) 226: 639, 1970.
24. Dobbing, J., and J. Sands. Quantitative growth and development of human brain. *Arch. Dis. Child.* 48: 757, 1973.
25. Dobbing, J., and E. M. Widdowson. The effect of undernutrition and subsequent rehabilitation on myelination of rat brain as measured by its composition. *Brain* 88: 357, 1965.
26. Fraňková, S., and R. H. Barnes. Influence of malnutrition in early life on exploratory behavior of rats. *J. Nutr.* 96: 477, 1968.
27. Fraňková, S., and R. H. Barnes. Effect of malnutrition in early life on avoidance conditioning and behavior of adult rats. *J. Nutr.* 96: 485, 1968.
28. Habicht, J- P., C. Yarbrough, A. Lechtig, and R. E. Klein. Relationships of birth weight, maternal nutrition, and infant mortality. *Nutr. Reports Internat.* 7: 533, 1973.
29. Hall, S. M., and F. J. Zeman. Kidney function of the progeny of rats fed a low protein diet. *J. Nutr.* 95: 49, 1968.
30. Holloway, R. L. The evolution of the primate brain: Some aspects of quantitative relations. *Brain Res.* 7: 121, 1968.
31. Hsueh, A. M., C. E. Augustin, and B. F. Chow. Growth of young rats after differential manipulation of maternal diet. *J. Nutr.* 91: 195, 1967.
32. Hunt, R. K., and M. Jacobson. Brain enhancement in tadpoles: Increased DNA concentration after somatotrophin or prolactin. *Science* 170: 342, 1970.
33. Lee, C. J., and B. F. Chow. Metabolism of proteins by progeny of underfed mother rats. *J. Nutr.* 94: 20, 1968.
34. Levitsky, D. A., and R. H. Barnes. The behavioral effects of early protein-calorie restriction in the adult rat. *Fed. Proc.* 28: 555, 1969.
35. Levitsky, D. A., and R. H. Barnes. Effect of early malnutrition on the reaction of adult rats to aversive stimuli. *Nature* 225: 468, 1970.
36. McKeown, T., and R. G. Record. Observations on foetal growth in multiple pregnancy in man. *J. Endocri.* 8: 386, 1952.
37. McKeown, T., and R. G. Record. The influence of placental size on foetal growth in man, with special reference to multiple pregnancy. *J. Endocri.* 9: 418, 1953.

38. McLaren, A. Genetic and environmental effects on foetal and placental growth in mice. *J. Reprod. Fertil.* 9: 79, 1965.

39. Ounsted, M. Familial factors affecting fetal growth. In *Prenatal Factors Affecting Human Development*, Pan Amer. Health Organization, Scientific Publ. No. 185, Washington, D.C., 1969, p. 60.

40. Picon, L. Effect of insulin on growth and biochemical composition of the rat fetus. *Endocri.* 81: 1419, 1967.

41. Stephan, J. K., B. Chow, L. A. Frohman, and B. F. Chow. Relationship of growth hormone to the growth retardation associated with maternal dietary restriction. *J. Nutr.* 101: 1453, 1971.

42. van Marthens, E., L. Grauel, and S. Zamenhof. Enhancement of prenatal development by operative restriction of litter size in the rabbit. *Life Sci.* 11 (Part I): 1031, 1972.

43. van Marthens, E., L. Grauel, and S. Zamenhof. Enhancement of prenatal development in the rat by operative restriction of litter size. *Biol. Neonate* 25: 53, 1974.

44. van Marthens, E., S. Harel, and S. Zamenhof. Experimental intrauterine growth retardation: A new animal model for the study of altered brain development. *Biol. Neonate* 26: 221, 1975.

45. van Marthens, E., and S. Zamenhof. Deoxyribonucleic acid of neonatal rat cerebrum increased by operative restriction of litter size. *Exp. Neurol.* 23: 214, 1969.

46. Walker, W. I., J. I. Johnson, and B. H. Pubols, Jr. Some morphological and physiological characteristics of the somatic sensory systems in raccoons. *Am. Zool.* 4: 75, 1964.

47. Warden, C. J., S. Ross, and S. Zamenhof. The effect of artificial changes in the brain on maze-learning in the white rat. *Science* 95: 414, 1942.

48. Wigglesworth, J. S. Experimental growth retardation in the foetal rat. *J. Path. Bact.* 88: 1, 1964.

49. Williams, R. J. "Supernutrition" as a strategy for the control of disease. *Proc. Natl. Acad. Sci.* 68: 2899a, 1971.

50. Winick, M. Malnutrition and brain development. *J. Pediat.* 74: 667, 1969.

51. Winick, M. Cellular growth in intrauterine malnutrition. *Pediat. Clin. N. Am.* 17: 69, 1970.

52. Winick, M. Malnutrition and intrauterine growth. *Nutr. Reports Internat.* 4: 239, 1971.

53. Winick, M., and A. Noble. Quantitative changes in DNA, RNA and protein during prenatal and postnatal growth in the rat. *Devel. Biol.* 12: 451, 1965.

54. Winick, M., and A. Noble. Cellular response during malnutrition at various ages. *J. Nutr.* 89: 300, 1966.

55. Winick, M., and A. Noble. Cellular response with increased feeding in neonatal rats. *J. Nutr.* 91: 179, 1967.

Stephen Zamenhof and Edith van Marthens

56. Winick, M., and P. Rosso. Head circumference and cellular growth of the brain in normal and marasmic children. *J. Pediat.* 74: 774, 1969.
57. Zamenhof, S. Stimulation of the proliferation of neurons by the growth hormone. I. Experiments on tadpoles. *Growth* 5: 123, 1941.
58. Zamenhof, S. Stimulation of cortical-cell proliferation by the growth hormone. III. Experiments on albino rats. *Physiol. Zool.* 15: 281, 1942.
59. Zamenhof, S. Studies on some factors influencing cell number in prenatal brain. In *Prenatal Factors Affecting Human Development,* Pan Amer. Health Organization, Scientific Publ. No. 185, Washington, D.C., 1969, p. 19.
60. Zamenhof, S., H. Bursztyn, K. Rich, and P. J. Zamenhof. The determination of deoxyribonucleic acid (DNA) and of cell number in brain. *J. Neurochem.* 11: 505, 1964.
61. Zamenhof, S., L. Grauel, and E. van Marthens. Study of possible correlations between prenatal brain development and placental weight. *Biol. Neonate* 18: 140, 1971.
62. Zamenhof, S., L. Grauel, E. van Marthens, and R. A. Stillinger. Quantitative determination of DNA in preserved brains and brain sections. *J. Neurochem.* 19: 61, 1972.
63. Zamenhof, S., D. Guthrie, and D. Clarkson. Study of possible correlations between body weights and brain parameters in neonatal and mature rats. *Biol. Neonate* 24: 354, 1974.
64. Zamenhof, S., S. M. Hall, L. Grauel, E. van Marthens, and M. J. Donahue. Deprivation of amino acids and prenatal brain development in rats. *J. Nutr.* 104: 1002, 1974.
65. Zamenhof, S., and G. B. Holzman. Study of correlations between head circumferences, placental parameters and neonatal body weights. *Obstet. Gyn.* 41: 855, 1973.
66. Zamenhof, S., and E. van Marthens. Hormonal and nutritional aspects of prenatal brain development. In *Cellular Aspects of Neural Growth and Differentiation,* D. C. Pease, ed., UCLA Forum in Medical Sciences, No. 14, Univ. of California Press, Berkeley, 1971, p. 329.
67. Zamenhof, S., and E. van Marthens. Study of factors influencing prenatal brain development. *Molec. Cell. Biochem.* 4: 157, 1974.
68. Zamenhof, S., E. van Marthens, and H. Bursztyn. The effect of hormones on DNA synthesis and cell number in the developing chick and rat brain. In *Hormones in Development,* M. Hamburgh and E. J. W. Barrington, eds., Appleton, New York, 1971, p. 101.
69. Zamenhof, S., E. van Marthens, and L. Grauel. DNA (cell number) and protein in neonatal rat brain: Alteration by timing maternal dietary protein restriction. *J. Nutr.* 101: 1265, 1971.
70. Zamenhof, S., E. van Marthens, and L. Grauel. DNA (cell number) in neonatal brain: Alteration by maternal dietary caloric restriction. *Nutr. Reports Internat.* 4: 269, 1971.

76

71. Zamenhof, S., E. van Marthens, and L. Grauel. Prenatal cerebral development in nutritionally restricted animals: Rehabilitation by treatment with growth hormone. *Science* 174: 954, 1971.

72. Zamenhof, S., E. van Marthens, and L. Grauel. DNA (cell number) in neonatal brain: Second generation (F_2) alteration by maternal (F_0) dietary protein restriction. *Science* 172: 850, 1971.

73. Zamenhof, S., E. van Marthens, and L. Grauel. DNA (cell number) and protein in rat brain. *Nutr. Metab.* 14: 262, 1972.

74. Zamenhof, S., E. van Marthens, and L. Grauel. Studies on some factors influencing prenatal brain development. *In Regulation of Organ and Tissue Growth*, R. J. Goss, ed., Academic Press, New York, 1972, p. 41.

75. Zamenhof, S., E. van Marthens, and F. L. Margolis. DNA (cell number) and protein in neonatal brain: Alteration by maternal dietary restriction. *Science* 160: 322, 1968.

76. Zeman, F. J. Effect on the young rat of maternal protein restriction. *J. Nutr.* 93: 167, 1967.

77. Zeman, F. J., and E. C. Stanbrough. Effect of maternal protein deficiency on cellular development in the fetal rat. *J. Nutr.* 99: 274, 1969.

John D. Fernstrom and Loy D. Lytle **6**

Long-term Consumption of Low-protein Corn-based Diets: Effect on Serotonin Synthesis in Rat Brain, and on Sensitivity to Painful Stimuli

Introduction

Malnutrition, both experimental and clinical, has been associated with altered brain composition and impaired mental function. Severe dietary restrictions have lead to reduced brain size, cell number, protein and lipid content, and poor performance on intelligence, and sensory and motor function tests.

Neuronal communications in the brain and, ultimately, brain function, depend on the presence and proper functioning of a class of compounds termed neurotransmitters. These chemicals are released from nerves following depolarization, and elicit the depolarization of immediately adjacent neurons, thus propagating nerve impulses. To date, all of the known neurotransmitters are low-molecular-weight compounds; most are either simple metabolites of amino acids (serotonin, norepinephrine, dopamine, epinephrine), or amino acids themselves (for example, gamma amino butyric acid [GABA], glycine, aspartate). Altering the synthesis, storage, release, or metabolism of neurotransmitters can have profound physiological and behavioral consequences.

The changes in mental function and behavior that accompany malnutrition may be the result of diet-induced changes in neurotransmitter function, although little direct evidence for this hypothesis has been provided in the past. This seems particularly surprising in view of the metabolic relationship of neurotransmitters and amino acids. It seems very plausible, for example, that restrictions in the intake of amino acids, particularly of essential amino acids that are neurotransmitter precursors, might ultimately reduce transmitter synthesis by limiting substrate availability. Similarly, reduced protein synthesis in brain associated with malnutrition might decrease the concentrations of brain neurotransmitters by reducing the amounts of the enzymes involved in the synthesis of these compounds.

We have been interested in a particular model of malnutrition, that resulting from the chronic ingestion of a corn-based diet. Corn was selected as the dietary protein source because of its very low tryptophan content; we suspected that dietary tryptophan restriction might ultimately limit the synthesis in brain of a particular neurotransmitter, serotonin (5-HT), that derives from this essential amino acid. The ingestion of this diet by rats for relatively short periods (6 weeks) depresses brain serotonin levels; in addition, these changes are associated with an alteration in a particular behavioral response thought to be controlled at least in part by serotonergic neurons: pain sensitivity. Animals consuming the corn diet become extremely sensitive to painful stimuli. Further supporting the role of serotonin in pain sensitivity were our studies showing that in corn-malnourished rats, normal sensitivity to pain could be restored by simple pharmacologic techniques that rapidly raise brain serotonin, or by the addition of tryptophan to the diet (either as casein, or as the free amino acid).

Our studies thus show, for the first time, that reducing the intake of normal dietary constituents can lead to a depression in the brain levels of a specific neurotransmitter, serotonin, which can be associated with a deficit in a particular brain function, pain sensitivity, known to be controlled in part by serotonergic neurons. Hence, it seems likely that at least some of the mental and behavioral dysfunctions associated with malnutrition *are* related specifically to altered neurotransmission secondary to transmitter deficiencies.

Chronic, Diet-induced Changes in Brain Serotonin Levels and Synthesis

Among the earliest investigators to demonstrate that brain serotonin levels could be depressed by the chronic restriction of tryptophan in the diet were Zbinden and his associates.[19] They found that the brains of rats and mice fed a tryptophan-deficient synthetic diet for 2 to 4 weeks contained 40 to 50 percent less serotonin than the brains of well-nourished control animals. Simi-

79

lar results were obtained by Gal et al.,[10] Gal and Drewes,[9] Culley et al.,[3] and Thomas and Wysor,[17] who used diets containing acid-hydrolysates of casein *in lieu* of the protein itself (acid hydrolysis of casein produces a mixture of amino acids similar to that in the intact protein, but deficient in tryptophan due to its destruction during hydrolysis). Boullin[1] further confirmed these findings, using synthetic amino acid diets lacking in tryptophan.

The decrease in serotonin in the brains of tryptophan-deprived rats was accompanied by reductions in brain norepinephrine, and was associated with convulsions and ataxia in rats whose brains contained less than 20 percent of normal brain serotonin levels. Thomas and Wysor[17] observed that the decrease in brain serotonin would not occur unless animals were given niacin supplements to block the development of pellagra. The reductions in brain serotonin were unaffected by the addition of sulfasuccidine to the diet, and thus were independent of tryptophan metabolism by intestinal flora.

Wang et al.[18] and Green et al.[11] independently demonstrated that brain serotonin levels could also be *increased* by chronically feeding rats diets supplemented with tryptophan (1.1 percent). Thus, the correlation between dietary tryptophan content and brain serotonin concentration held over a rather wide range of dietary tryptophan levels that were both above and below normal values.

Serum tryptophan concentrations were measured in only one of the above studies, and were found to fall substantially within 4 days after rats began ingesting a tryptophan-deficient diet. No data were obtained on the effects of these diets on brain tryptophan concentrations, and thus no conclusions could be drawn as to whether brain serotonin levels changed specifically in response to alterations in substrate (i.e., tryptophan) availability to the brain. It seems equally likely, for example, that brain serotonin levels might fall in response to reductions in the activities of serotonin-synthesizing enzymes secondary to a decrease in brain protein synthesis (rats ingesting such diets usually show signs of malnutrition), or in response to a decline in the ability of serotonin-containing neurons in the brain to store the amine.

As a first step toward understanding the mechanism(s) by which chronic ingestion of a tryptophan-deficient diet reduces brain serotonin levels, we have measured blood and brain tryptophan, and brain serotonin levels in young rats that consumed for 6 weeks a diet containing corn as the only source of protein.[7] Corn was selected as the dietary amino acid source for these studies because its protein (principally maize) is tryptophan-deficient, and because corn is a principal source of protein in several human subpopulations.

By the end of the 6-week period, rats ingesting the corn diet had increased their body weights by only 40 to 50 percent, as had animals consuming two other diets that were pair-fed to the consumption of the corn-fed rats (these other diets contained either 6 percent casein, or corn supplemented with L-tryptophan, 0.1 percent dry weight). In contrast, animals in a fourth diet group ingesting 18 percent casein *ad libitum* for 6 weeks increased their body weights by about 270 percent. The relatively small weight gains of the corn- and 6 percent casein-fed animals can be explained at least in part by the lower total daily food intake of these rats, compared to that of rats ingesting the 18 percent casein diet (about 8.5 gr/day versus 13.5 gr/day, respectively).

Rats ingesting the corn diet consumed only about 10 percent of the tryptophan of those consuming 18 percent casein. In these "corn-fed" animals, plasma tryptophan concentrations were 27 percent, brain tryptophan levels 40 percent, and brain serotonin 62 percent of the values in rats ingesting 18 percent casein. If, instead of the standard corn diet, rats consumed the corn diet containing 0.1 percent L-tryptophan (100 mg/100 gr of diet, dry weight), the levels of tryptophan in plasma and brain and of serotonin in brain were all significantly greater than those in rats ingesting the unsupplemented corn diet. In animals ingesting 6 percent casein, that provided them with approximately 40 percent more tryptophan each day than that consumed by corn-fed rats, plasma and brain tryptophan levels were also elevated significantly over those of corn-fed rats. Brain serotonin contents were also higher, but the increase was not statistically significant.

These findings, using a natural protein as the dietary source of amino acids, support the notion that long-term reductions in the tryptophan content of the diet are associated with depressed levels of serotonin in the brain and with reductions in the plasma and brain concentrations of tryptophan. This hypothesis is best supported by our observations that animals ingesting the 0.1 percent tryptophan-supplemented corn diet have significantly greater amounts of tryptophan in their plasmas and brains, and serotonin in their brains, than do rats ingesting the unsupplemented corn diet.

Our results suggest a causal relationship between plasma and brain tryptophan levels, and brain serotonin concentrations. It is possible, however, that the reduced serotonin content in the brains of the corn-fed rats might not have resulted from decreased synthesis of the amine secondary to a limitation on substrate availability. Equally likely factors that might have precipitated the depression in brain serotonin in corn-malnourished rats include: (1) a decrease in the number of serotonin-synthesizing neurons in brain, (2) a reduction in the activity of the enzymes involved in serotonin biosynthesis, (3) an acceleration in serotonin metabolism, or (4) an impairment in serotonin storage or reuptake.

We have initiated further studies to elucidate the factors contributing to the reduction in brain 5-HT in corn-malnourished rats by attempting to elevate brain 5-HT and 5-hydroxyindole acetic acid (5-HIAA) levels acutely in these animals with a single injection of L-tryptophan. A rapid rise in 5-HT and 5-HIAA would provide evidence that defects in the neurochemical machinery for serotonin synthesis and storage probably are not primarily responsible for the low brain serotonin content, and that the deficiency in substrate is an important contributor to the reduced indole content.

Groups of rats, fed either the corn diet (low tryptophan) or an 18 percent casein diet for 6 weeks, received an intraperitoneal injection of L-tryptophan (25, 50, 100 mg/kg), and were killed one hour later. As shown in Figure 6.1, each dose caused greater increases in brain tryptophan concentrations in corn-fed rats than in casein-fed animals, even though serum tryptophan concentrations were always greater in the casein-fed animals. The 50- and 100-mg/kg doses were associated with higher brain tryptophan concentrations in corn-fed than in casein-fed rats. Tryptophan injection elevated brain 5-hydroxyindole contents in both diet groups (Table 6.1); at each dose tested, brain 5-HIAA usually increased to a greater extent than 5-HT, regardless of diet.

Although the increases in brain tryptophan concentration were not perfectly dose-related, the changes in brain 5-hydroxyindole levels always paralleled the changes in brain tryptophan. Thus, in corn-fed rats, the 100-mg/kg dose failed to elevate either brain tryptophan or brain 5-hydroxyindoles over values obtained from

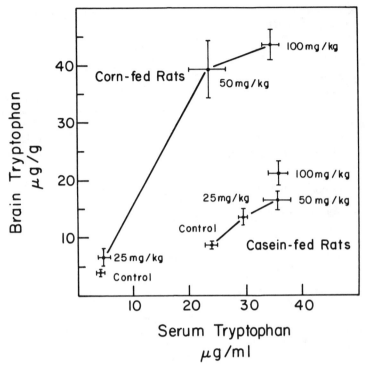

Figure 6.1. Dose-response relationship between serum and brain tryptophan in corn-fed, and casein-fed rats injected with various doses of L-tryptophan. Groups of 4 rats were killed 1 hour after the intraperitoneal injection of L-tryptophan (0, 25, 50, or 100 mg/kg). Data are presented as the mean ± S.E. From J. D. Fernstrom and M. J. Hirsch, *Life Sci.* 17: 455, 1975.

animals receiving the 50-mg/kg dose (Table 6.1). Similarly, in casein-fed rats, the 50-mg/kg dose elevated neither brain constituent above the levels observed in animals injected with the 25-mg/kg dose (Table 6.1).

A given dose of tryptophan tended to cause greater increments in brain tryptophan in corn-fed than in casein-fed rats (Figure 6.1). To determine whether this tendency might have resulted from differences in brain tryptophan uptake, we measured the concentrations of 5 neutral amino acids known to compete with tryptophan for brain uptake (tyrosine, phenylalanine, leucine, isoleucine, and valine) in sera obtained from uninjected corn- and

Table 6.1. The effect of various doses of L-tryptophan on brain tryptophan and 5-hydroxyindoles in rats consuming the corn or casein diets*

Tryptophan dose	Brain			
	Tryptophan	5-HT	5-HIAA	(5-HT + 5-HIAA)
	μg/g	ng/brain	ng/brain	nM/brain
Control				
Corn-fed	3.52 ± 0.19	345 ± 40	480 ± 20	4.26 ± 0.42
Casein-fed	8.61 ± 0.23	641 ± 55	926 ± 23	7.78 ± 0.47
25 mg/kg				
Corn-fed	6.98 ± 1.12	567 ± 53	895 ± 63	8.13 ± 0.44
Casein-fed	13.00 ± 1.26	749 ± 41	1755 ± 60	13.43 ± 0.49
50 mg/kg				
Corn-fed	38.26 ± 6.27	755 ± 19	1778 ± 31	13.58 ± 0.25
Casein-fed	15.86 ± 2.29	721 ± 24	1680 ± 72	12.66 ± 0.44
100 mg/kg				
Corn-fed	43.30 ± 2.54	551 ± 54	1683 ± 128	12.47 ± 0.72
Casein-fed	21.40 ± 2.61	786 ± 17	2230 ± 71	16.13 ± 0.45

*Data are from the same animals as described in Figure 6.1. By a two-way analysis of variance, very highly significant differences ($P < 0.001$) were generated in brain tryptophan, 5-HT, and (5-HT + 5-HIAA) by diet or by tryptophan injection. Moreover, there was a highly significant difference generated by the interaction of diet and tryptophan administration. Data are presented as mean ± S.E.

casein-fed rats. The serum concentrations of each of these amino acids was substantially less in corn-fed than in casein-fed animals (Table 6.2). We also measured the concentrations of serum-free tryptophan in both diet groups, inasmuch as several investigators have suggested that brain tryptophan levels are controlled by the proportion of the amino acid in serum that is not bound to albumin.[12,15] As shown in Table 6.3, serum total tryptophan was depressed in corn-fed rats; the serum-free tryptophan level also decreased, but proportionally less than total tryptophan. Consequently, the *percent* of total amino acid present in the unbound moiety increased, from 16.1 percent to 27.4 percent (Table 6.3). This effect may be explained by the large decrease in serum albumin concentrations (Table 6.3); nonesterified fatty-acid levels were almost identical in the two groups, and thus cannot account for the difference in the percent of tryptophan bound to albumin.

From this data, it is not possible to conclude whether the much

Table 6.2. Concentrations of branched-chain and aromatic amino acids in the sera of rats fed either the corn or casein diet for six weeks*

Amino acid	Casein-fed rats (nM/ml)	Corn-fed rats (nM/ml)
Tyrosine	136.48 ± 13.56	28.00 ± 2.31
Phenylalanine	71.88 ± 3.15	42.68 ± 1.82
Leucine	146.70 ± 2.60	99.98 ± 4.51
Isoleucine	100.54 ± 3.12	38.80 ± 1.11
Valine	189.32 ± 15.08	71.62 ± 3.82

*Groups of 5 rats were fed either the corn or the casein diet for 6 weeks. They were then killed in the morning, and their sera analyzed for neutral amino acid content. Data are presented as the mean ± S.E.; the concentration of each amino acid in corn-fed rats is significantly lower than that in casein-fed rats ($P < 0.001$).

larger increments in brain tryptophan that occur in corn-fed rats following tryptophan injection reflect primarily the low serum levels of competing neutral amino acids, or the reduced binding of tryptophan to serum albumin. However, other studies, performed in our laboratories over the past several years, support the notion that neutral amino acid competition for brain uptake is a much more important determinant of brain tryptophan levels than the binding of tryptophan to albumin in blood.

Table 6.3. The effect of corn malnutrition on serum albumin, nonesterified fatty acid, and free and bound tryptophan concentrations in rats*

Compound	Diet	
	Corn	Casein (18%)
Serum tryptophan		
Total (μg/ml)	4.0 ± 0.4†	24.2 ± 1.7
Free (μg/ml)	1.1 ± 0.2†	3.9 ± 0.1
Free (%)	27.4 ± 3.1†	16.1 ± 1.1
Serum NEFA (μeq/1)	0.27 ± 0.01	0.28 ± 0.03
Serum albumin (g/100 ml)	1.3 ± 0.1†	4.4 ± 0.3

*Groups of 5 corn-fed and casein-fed rats were killed in the morning. Blood was collected from the cervical wound and centrifuged. The sera were frozen until assay under 95 percent N_2 and 5 percent CO_2. Data are presented as the mean ± SE.
†$P < 0.005$ compared with 18 percent casein values.

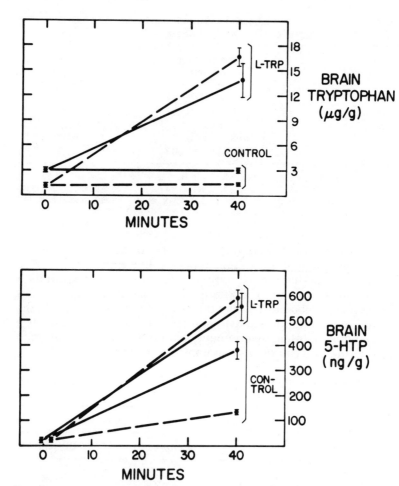

Figure 6.2. 5-Hydroxytryptophan accumulation in rat brain after the injection of RO4-4602 (800 mg/kg), an inhibitor of aromatic-L-amino acid decarboxylase. Upper panel: Brain tryptophan concentrations in corn- and casein-fed rats injected with RO4-4602, followed 10 minutes later by a second injection of saline or L-tryptophan (50 mg/kg). Data are presented as the mean ± S.E. Lower panel: Brain 5-hydroxytryptophan (5-HTP) levels in corn- and casein-fed rats injected with RO4-4602, followed by tryptophan or saline. Data are presented as the mean ± S.E. Dashed lines, corn-fed rats; solid lines, casein-fed rats. From J. D. Fernstrom and M. J. Hirsch, *J. Neurochem.* 28(4): 877, 1977.

Recently, we have estimated the rate of serotonin synthesis in corn-fed rats injected with tryptophan or its vehicle (Figure 6.2). The method employed is that of Carlsson et al.[2] which measures the accumulation of 5-hydroxytryptophan (5-HTP) following inhibition of aromatic L-amino acid decarboxylase with R04-4602. (Hence, this method estimates tryptophan hydroxylation *in vivo*, which is thought to be the rate-limiting reaction in serotonin synthesis: the rate of hydroxylation determines the overall rate of serotonin formation.) As indicated in Figure 6.2, untreated corn-fed rats synthesize much less 5-HTP than do well-nourished casein-fed rats. However, following tryptophan injection, the rate of 5-HTP formation is stimulated in both groups, so that 5-HTP accumulation appears identical in the two dietary groups. These data thus support the notion that the reduction in 5-HT levels in corn-fed rats is at least partly due to diminished synthesis of the amine, secondary to decreased substrate availability.

Chronic, Diet-induced Changes in Brain Serotonin Levels and Their Relationship to Behavior

Surgical and pharmacological manipulations that modify brain serotonin levels elicit changes in a variety of behavioral states, including sleep, locomotor activity, and the response to painful stimuli. For example, Tenen[16] and Fibiger et al.[8] showed that reductions in brain serotonin following the administration of parachlorophenylalanine, an inhibitor of tryptophan hydroxylase, increased the sensitivity to painful stimuli. Similarly, hyperalgesia and decreased forebrain serotonin levels are also observed in rats following electrolytic lesions that destroy the medial forebrain bundle, the septal nuclei, or the nucleus accumbens. The hyperalgesia and reduced concentrations of forebrain serotonin can be reversed in these animals by the injection of 5-hydroxytryptophan.

If the relationship between brain serotonin levels and changes in the response thresholds to painful stimuli are real, and not simply a chance correlation, then it should be possible to demonstrate alterations in pain sensitivity in animals receiving any treatment that modifies brain serotonin. Brain serotonin levels are substantially reduced in rats consuming for 6 weeks a diet containing corn as the only source of protein. To test the hypothesis that this dietary manipulation, by altering brain serotonin, might also change the response thresholds to painful stimuli, groups of

87

corn-fed and casein-fed rats were tested for their responses to electric foot shock at various intervals after institution of the diets. We used the flinch-jump method of W. O. Evans[4] to measure the response to pain. Briefly, animals were placed in the testing apparatus during the light portion of the day-night cycle, and given 6 alternating ascending and descending series of 10 shocks. With the onset of each shock presentation, animals were observed for the occurrence of a flinch response (a startle or crouching response in which all four paws remained in contact with the grid floor) or a jump response (a response in which the hind paws leave the grid floor simultaneously with the onset of the shock). Shock threshold intensities were determined for the flinch and the jump response, and were operationally defined as those shock intensities that elicited a flinch or a jump response 50 percent of the time.

Whereas the shock intensity necessary to elicit a flinch or a jump response in animals fed the 18 percent casein diet increased only slightly over the 14-week testing period, animals fed the tryptophan-poor diet showed flinch and jump response thresholds approximately half those of the control group within 2 weeks after exposure to the diet (Figure 6.3). In confirmation of our previous findings, the brains of animals fed the corn diet contained very low levels of tryptophan and serotonin. The results of this initial experiment suggested that dietary manipulations that affect the levels of serotonin in brain are associated with profound alterations in behavior.[13]

The reductions in brain tryptophan and serotonin that occur following the chronic consumption of the tryptophan-poor corn diet can be reversed within 3 to 4 days by giving the animals free access to diets that contain balanced concentrations of amino acids and adequate amounts of protein. To determine the extent to which the changes in response thresholds to electric shock might also be reversed as a function of dietary rehabilitation, groups of animals fed the corn diet for 10 weeks were offered a normal 18 percent casein diet. As indicated in Figure 6.3, the flinch and jump response thresholds returned to normal within 2 weeks after exposure to the normal diet. The behavioral rehabilitation produced by feeding animals the normal diet was correlated temporally with a return to normal of brain tryptophan and serotonin concentrations in these animals.[14]

The corn diet, while deficient in tryptophan (it contains 12

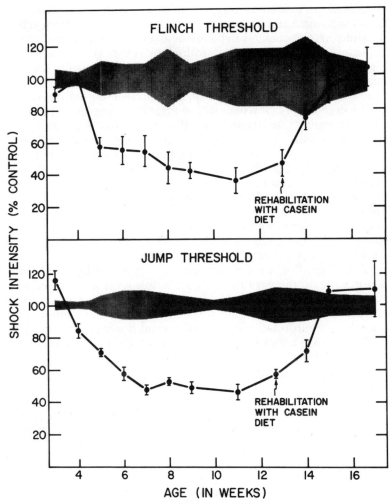

Figure 6.3. The effect of corn malnutrition on pain sensitivity. Groups of rats ingested the corn diet (filled circles and solid lines) or the casein diet (shaded areas) from the third to the thirteenth postnatal weeks. Thereafter, corn-fed rats were rehabilitated with the casein diet. All values are means ± S.E., in percents of casein-fed rat flinch and jump thresholds. From L. D. Lytle, R. B. Messing, L. Fisher, and L. Phebus, *Science* 190: 692, 1975.

percent of the amount of tryptophan in the casein diet), also contains inadequate amounts of protein (about 7 percent). Hence, it is possible that the changes in behavior associated with chronic corn ingestion, and their reversal following rehabilitation with the high-quality casein diet, may represent changes related to the protein content of the diet, rather than simply to the tryptophan concentration. To test this possibility, we switched rats malnourished on the corn diet for 9 weeks to a similar diet supplemented with normal amounts of tryptophan (the tryptophan-supplemented corn diet is still a low-protein diet). As can be seen in Table 6.4, after 4 weeks on this new diet, the jump response thresholds of animals fed the corn diet supplemented with tryptophan returned to normal. In addition, the consumption of this diet also returned the concentrations of brain serotonin and 5-HIAA to normal. These data indicate that the behavioral and biochemical changes in animals consuming the corn diet are related specifically to the effects of the diet on brain serotonin, and are not the result of the consumption of a diet deficient in protein.

In other studies, we determined the extent to which an acute, pharmacologic increase in brain serotonin level in corn-fed animals would restore the response thresholds to electric shock to normal values. Groups of rats placed on the corn or casein diet for 5 weeks were injected with one of several doses of L-tryptophan (0, 62.5, 125, or 250 mg/kg). Pain sensitivity thresholds, deter-

Table 6.4. Effects of different diets on brain 5-hydroxyindoles and on the electroshock jump threshold*

Diet	Jump threshold (ma)	Brain 5-HT (μg/g)	Brain 5-HIAA (μg/g)
Casein	.88 ± .06	.44 ± .01	.50 ± .01
Corn	.41 ± .01†	.27 ± .01†	.21 ± .01†
Corn + tryptophan	.73 ± .04‡	.46 ± .01‡	.48 ± .03‡

*Weanling albino rats were given *ad libitum* access to a tryptophan-poor corn diet, or to the 18 percent casein control diet beginning at 21 days of age. Nine weeks later, half of the corn-fed animals were given access to the corn diet supplemented with L-tryptophan (1.64 mg/kg dry weight). Four weeks later, animals were tested for their responses to electric shock, or were killed for biochemical assays. All values are the means ± S.E. (N = 8).

†p < .001 compared to casein-fed control group.

‡Not statistically different from casein-fed control group.

Table 6.5. Effect of L-tryptophan injection on electroshock sensitivity in rats consuming corn or casein diets*

Tryptophan dose	Shock intensity†	
	Corn diet	Casein diet
Vehicle	0.43 ± 0.02	0.85 ± 0.05
62.5 mg/kg	0.54 ± 0.06	0.95 ± 0.04
125 mg/kg	0.69 ± 0.02‡	0.78 ± 0.06
250 mg/kg	0.63 ± 0.04‡	0.88 ± 0.04

*Groups of rats were fed either the corn-based or casein-based diet for 6 weeks. At the end of this period, they were fasted overnight, and then injected (in groups of 8) with L-tryptophan or vehicle. Shock intensities were determined 1 hour later. Data are presented as the mean ± SEM.

†Shock intensity for jump response, in milliamperes.

‡P < 0.01 compared with appropriate vehicle-injected control group.

mined 1 hour later, increased in a dose-related manner in corn-fed rats, but not in animals consuming the normal diet (Table 6.5). This acute reversal of the hyperalgesia in corn-fed rats by the injection of tryptophan appears to be related to the specific effects of the amino acid on brain serotonin: large doses of l-dopa, the immediate precursor of the catecholamine neurotransmitters, have no effect on brain 5-HT or the jump threshold.

Summary

The consumption for 6 weeks of a diet containing corn as the only source of protein reduces serotonin levels in rat brain. The deficiency can be reversed *chronically* by feeding these animals a high-quality casein diet (18 percent), or the corn diet supplemented with L-tryptophan, or *acutely* by injecting the amino acid. The acute elevation of brain serotonin in corn-fed rats following tryptophan injection reflects stimulation of amine synthesis.

Corn-fed rats demonstrate a hypersensitivity to painful stimuli, a behavior thought to be related to the activity of serotonergic neurons in brain. In support of this relationship, the hyperalgesia can be reversed chronically by feeding animals diets adequate in tryptophan, or acutely by injecting them with replacement doses of the amino acid.

We are presently attempting to identify other behavioral changes, induced by chronic ingestion of the corn diet, that might be responsive to chronic or acute tryptophan administration.

References

1. Boullin, D. J. Behavior of rats depleted of 5-hydroxytryptamine by feeding a diet free of tryptophan. *Psychopharmacologia* 5: 28, 1963.
2. Carlsson, A., W. Kehr, M. Lindqvist, T. Magnussen, and C. V. Atack. Regulation of monoamine metabolism in the central nervous system. *Pharmacol. Rev.* 24: 371, 1972.
3. Culley, W. J., R. N. Saunders, E. T. Mertz and D. H. Jolly. Effect of a tryptophan deficient diet on brain serotonin and plasma tryptophan level. *Proc. Soc. Exp. Biol. Med.* 113: 645–648, 1963.
4. Evans, W. O. A new technique for the investigation of some analgesic drugs on a reflexive behavior in the rat. *Psychopharmacologia* 2: 318, 1961.
5. Fernstrom, J. D., and M. J. Hirsch. Rapid repletion of brain serotonin in malnourished corn-fed rats following L-tryptophan injection. *Life Sci.* 17: 455, 1975.
6. Fernstrom, J. D., and M. J. Hirsch. Brain serotonin synthesis: Reduction in corn-malnourished rats. *J. Neurochem.* 28(4): 877, 1977.
7. Fernstrom, J. D., and R. J. Wurtman. Effect of chronic corn consumption on serotonin content of rat brain. *Nature New Biol.* 234: 62, 1971.
8. Fibiger, H. C., P. H. Mertz, and B. A. Campbell. The effect of p-chlorophenylalanine on aversion thresholds and reactivity to foot shock. *Physiol. Behav.* 8: 259, 1972.
9. Gal, E. M., and P. A. Drewes. Studies on the metabolism of 5-hydroxytryptamine (serotonin) effect of tryptophan deficiency in rats. *Proc. Soc. Exp. Biol. Med.* 110: 368, 1962.
10. Gal, E. M., P. A. Drewes, and C. A. Barraclough. Effect of reserpine and the metabolism of serotonin in tryptophan deficiency (rat). *Biochem. Pharmacol.* 8: 32, 1961.
11. Green, H., S. M. Greenberg, R. W. Erickson, J. L. Sawyer, and T. Ellison. Effect of dietary phenylalanine and tryptophan upon rat brain amine levels. *J. Pharmacol. Exp. Therap.* 136: 174–178, 1962.
12. Knott, P. J., and G. Curzon. Free tryptophan in plasma and brain tryptophan metabolism. *Nature* 239: 452, 1972.
13. Lytle, L. D., R. B. Messing, L. Fisher, and L. Phebus. Effects of long-term corn consumption on brain serotonin and the response to electric shock. *Science* 190: 692, 1975.
14. Messing, R. B., L. Fisher, L. Phebus, and L. Lytle. Interaction of diet and drugs in the regulation of brain 5-hydroxyindoles and the response to painful electric shock. *Life Sci.* 18: 707, 1976.

15. Tagliamonte, A., G. Biggio, and G. L. Gessa. Possible role of free plasma tryptophan in controlling brain tryptophan concentrations. *Riv. Pharmacol. Terapia* 2: 251, 1971.
16. Tenen, S. The effects of p-chlorophenylalanine, a serotonin depletor, on avoidance acquisition, pain sensitivity and related behavior in the rat. *Psychopharmacologia* 10: 204, 1967.
17. Thomas, R. G., and W. G. Wysor. Alteration of serotonin metabolism in rats deficient in niacin and tryptophan. *Proc. Soc. Exp. Biol. Med.* 126: 374, 1967.
18. Wang, H. L., V. H. Harwalker, and H. A. Waisman. Effect of dietary phenylalanine and tryptophan on brain serotonin. *Arch. Biochem. Biophys.* 96: 181, 1962.
19. Zbinden, G., A. Pletscher, and A. Studer. Effect of diet on chromaffin cells in the intestine and on the 5-hydroxytryptamine content of brain and intestine. *Z. ges Exp. Med.* 129: 615, 1958.

P. J. Morgane, O. Resnick, W. C. Stern, 7
W. B. Forbes, J. D. Bronzino, M. Miller,
J. P. Leahy, E. Hawrylewicz, and J. Kissane

Maternal Protein Malnutrition and the Developing Nervous System

For the past five years our group has been carrying out an interdisciplinary project studying the effects of maternal protein restriction on anatomical, neurophysiological, biochemical, and behavioral development in rats. Applying a variety of methodologies, we have studied ontogenetically many indicators of developing brain function in nutritionally deprived rats. One of the central dogmas of developmental neurobiology is implicit in the belief that structural maturation of neurons and synapses leads to an increasing capacity of the brain for complex physiological operations which result in progressively more elaborate behavioral activities of the developing organism. A corollary of this is the assumption that morphophysiology and behavior are sufficiently interrelated so that perturbations in morphophysiological development will influence or modify the development of behavior, and vice versa. It is our belief that in order to derive information about local brain abnormalities, such as biochemical pathology, the brain has to be studied by a battery of techniques. Since it is likely that many insults to the brain are not drastic and result in "minimal brain dysfunction," it is imperative that these be analyzed by application of electrographic, biochemical, anatomical, and behavioral approaches, each complementing the other and each with its own resolving power.

Electrophysiological Effects of Chronic Protein Malnutrition in the Rat

The objectives of our neurophysiological studies have been to analyze the ontogenetic development of several electrographic indicators of brain function in nutritionally deprived rats. These indices of brain malfunction in states of undernutrition and malnutrition may serve to localize the pathology, shed light on the primary nature of the disturbance, and provide prognostic information on the underlying pathology.

Quantitative analysis of *critical periods* in electrophysiological maturation of the brain is the most profitable way to utilize electro-ontogenetic indicators of delayed or perturbed development. Our overall aim has been to examine a series of electrographic indicators of maturational sequences as a means of evaluating the effects of protein malnutrition on electrical activity of the central nervous system. We have sought to determine critical periods of vulnerability of the developing brain and its recovery potential following reinstitution of adequate protein diets at birth and various periods up to weaning, and at different time periods in young and older adults. Each electrographic indicator provides valuable, complementary information regarding the sensitivity to insult of underlying brain mechanisms responsible for generating the electrical signals.

Our EEG studies of developing organisms have been primarily directed to the time and site of appearance of measurable gross potentials and also to the growth and differentiation of periodic patterns of these potentials in different brain areas. The EEG has markedly different kinds of appearance and differentiation of its components in the various areas of the brain, and, by studying the trends of this differentiation regionally, the temporal progression to "mature" EEG patterns can provide extremely valuable clues as to local brain dysfunction. These trends of differentiation have been especially brought out by analysis of the development of the various frequency components in the frequency histograms derived by computer techniques from brain EEG activity. We have concentrated on quantitative analysis of the developing EEG and are presently developing a power spectral atlas for quantitating electro-ontogenesis of the EEG in the rat brain at several ages which will serve as a baseline indicator for comparison with regional alterations seen in protein malnourished rats. We do not agree with John Dobbing's notation that electrophysiology might not have a significant role to play in defining abnormal brain function following nutritional insults. He mentions that electrophysiology may not be useful as a "horoscope" or for the detection of "criminality," and we would fully agree with him on these extreme examples. The EEG is not an indicator of some specific global behaviors but, as we who work with the EEG can well testify, if properly used and quantitatively analyzed, it can serve as a powerful indicator of disturbed brain function. This is especially so if one has quantitative normal baseline data of electrographic function in given parts of the brain against which to compare the effects of insult. As is well known, the EEG serves best as a direct indicator of what we term the vigilance states, that is, waking, slow-wave sleep, and REM sleep. It also serves clinically to localize disturbed physiology, such as an epileptic focus, and so on.

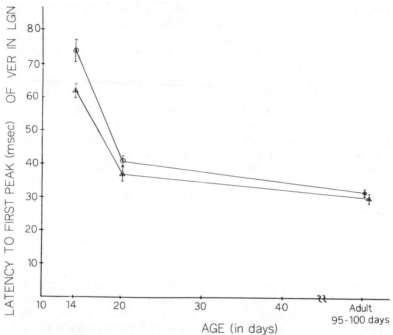

Figure 7.1. Mean (± SE) latencies of the first negative wave of the averaged visual evoked (flash) response obtained in the LGN at a flash frequency of 0.5 Hz. Significant differences exist between the latencies of the visual evoked response (VER) components in those animals reared on the 8 percent casein diet and those on the 25 percent casein diet at ages 14 and 20 days (n = 6 per time point). With progressing age the latencies to the first peak progressively merge so that by 95 to 100 days no differences in these values were seen. Circles represent 8 percent rats, triangles represent 25 percent rats. (From Bronzino et al., *Biol. Psychiat.* 10: 175–184, 1975.)

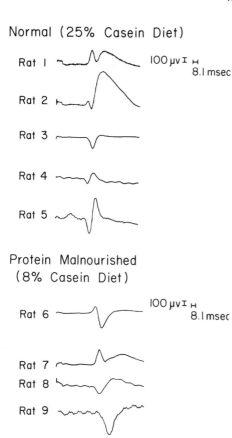

Normal (25% Casein Diet)

Rat 1
Rat 2
Rat 3
Rat 4
Rat 5

Protein Malnourished
(8% Casein Diet)

Rat 6
Rat 7
Rat 8
Rat 9

100 μv⊥ ⊢
8.1 msec

Figure 7.2. Averaged (256) visually evoked electrocortical responses (VER) obtained from nine 14-day-old rats. VER's obtained from the control group (25 percent casein diet) are shown in the top half of the figure, while those elicited from the protein-malnourished (8 percent casein diet) animals of the same age are displayed in the bottom half of the figure. The latencies to the first peak in the VER's of the protein-malnourished rats were significantly longer than in the normals. (From Bronzino et al., *Biol. Psychiat.* 10: 175–184, 1975.)

In our studies we have stressed that the spontaneous EEG can yield basic information concerning the degree of maturation of components of the central nervous system. In studying the developmental aspects of EEG activity in the rat it can be shown that there are apparently several critical periods in its development as evaluated by changes in the average EEG frequency. There is a critical period at approximately 9 days of age and a second critical period at approximately 15 days postnatally (the latter when the rats open their eyes). The EEG of the normal developing rat shows mostly adult characteristics and patterns at an age of 16 to 20 days.

We have been concentrating on analysis of the maturation of the

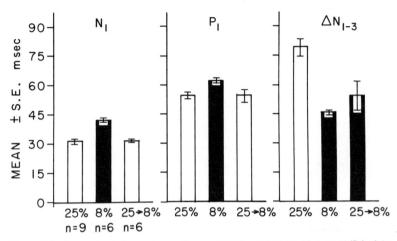

Figure 7.3. Latencies to the first negative peak (N_1) and first positive peak (P_1) of the visual evoked response in the lateral geniculate nucleus (LGN). Also shown is the interval of time between N_1 and N_3 (the third negative wave in the response) as indicated by ΔN_{1-3}. The first two bars for N_1, P_1, and ΔN_{1-3} are data from 20-day-old rats. Note that N_1 and P_1 are significantly delayed (longer latency to each of these waves following the light flash) in the 8 percent as compared to the 25 percent protein-fed animals. The third bar in each sequence shows that when adult (over 60-day-old) rats are reversed from a 25 percent diet to 8 percent diet for several weeks there is no effect on the latencies to wave N_1 or P_1 in the visual evoked response. (From Bronzino et al., *Biol. Psychiat.* 10: 175–184, 1975.)

EEG in the states of sleep and wakefulness. Ontogenesis of the sleep patterns, that is, the development of both the REM phase and the slow-wave sleep phase have received particular attention. The study of the sleep states or vigilance maturation relates to processes of attention, perception, and learning, and bears clear relationship to problems of mental retardation. We have also been studying evoked potential activity in both sensory and nonsensory systems, since an analysis of these potentials indicates the development of function in definable neural pathways. Abnormalities in the latency of appearance of individual waves, character of wave form, and nature of recovery characteristics of these component waves following insult to the nervous system serve as sensitive signs for specific insult in given neural pathways. We have studied evoked potential activity in sensory (visual system) and nonsensory systems (thalamocortical evoked response and the transcallosal evoked responses) and will review these briefly. The maturational sequence of visually evoked lateral geniculate or cortical responses elicited in the rat have been known for some time, and it has been long thought that neonatal undernutrition retards normal development of visual evoked responses during maturation. In our studies, however, we worked with a very specific type of undernutrition, that is, protein malnutrition, and studied the effects of this insult upon the maturation of the visual evoked response elicited in the lateral geniculate nucleus and in the visual cortex of the developing rat.[3] We showed that lateral geniculate and cortical visually evoked responses in all younger rats (normal and protein malnourished at 14 and 20 days of age) differed from those of older animals (95 to 100 days) as to latency, and time to the first positive and first negative components of the

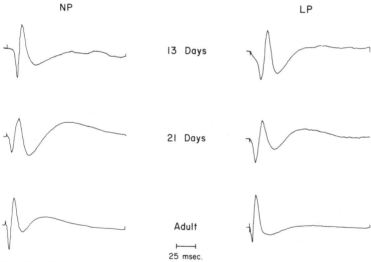

Figure 7.4. Representative examples of average of 16 trans-callosal evoked response at 13, 21, and 60 to 66 days of age in low-protein (LP) and normal protein (NP) animals. Ontogenic development in wave-form is essentially similar in the two groups. Differences in latency (average first 3 peaks) between LP and NP groups is obvious at day 13, but this difference disappears at 21 and 65 days of age even though animals were continued on the 8 percent protein diet. (From Forbes et al., Devel. Psychobiol. 8: 503–509, 1975.)

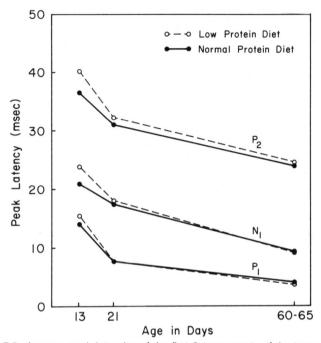

Figure 7.5. Average peak latencies of the first 3 components of the trans-callosal evoked response in low-protein (LP) and normal protein (NP) animals at age 13, 21, and 60 to 66 days. At the earliest age, peak latencies are greater in the LP group. The magnitude of the difference in latency at this age is greater for the later peaks than for the earliest peak, suggesting that the effect is not due simply to an initial transmission delay. At later ages, this effect is not seen despite the fact that the dietary (LP) treatments were continued. (From Forbes et al., *Devel. Psychobiol.* 8: 503–509, 1975.)

response (Figures 7.1 and 7.2). However, in addition to expected differences due to age or development, the protein-malnourished rats differed significantly from the normal group as to latency to first positive peak and first negative components in the younger age period, that is, up to day 20. No differences between the normal and protein-deprived group were noted in adult animals. Dietary reversal in the adult (from 25 to 8 percent protein) did not reinstitute latency differences in the appearance of the various peaks in the components of the visual evoked response (Figure 7.3). Thus, protein malnutrition during development appeared to retard the ontogenetic maturation of the visual system, and it appeared that even when the low-protein diet was maintained in the adult period there was a tendency for the visual evoked response to return to normal. Hence, we were likely dealing more with a delayed or *retarded* phenomena and not one that was permanently blocked by this type and degree of malnutrition.

In another study we examined the effects of chronic protein malnutrition on transcallosal evoked responses in the rat and found that the evoked response latency was significantly greater in malnourished animals at 13 days of age, whereas in adulthood no such latency differences were seen (Figures 7.4 and 7.5). Poststimulation excitability was not significantly affected by the dietary treatment. These results are in line with our findings of the effects of malnutrition on sensory (visual) evoked potentials. By avoiding the use of specific sensory stimulation, however, this study demonstrated the dietary effect upon ontogeny of cortical

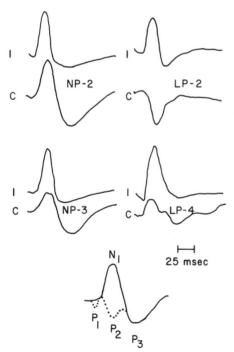

Figure 7.6. Effect of chronic dietary protein restriction on the rate and degree of incrementation of the cortical incremental response. Normalized response amplitude (N_1 to P_3 waves—see Figure 7.7) averaged across subjects in the normal protein-reared (control) and low protein-reared (8) percent groups are shown. One-second trains of stimuli were repeatedly presented. Within trains, stimulus repetition rates of 6, 8, and 10 pulses per second (PPS) were used. For both groups incrementation (waxing of response amplitude) is greatest under the 8 PPS condition. Differences between groups are not statistically significant.

P. J. Morgane et al.

evoked potentials independent of any possible effects on sensory receptor mechanisms.

We also studied thalamocortical evoked responses, that is, cortical incremental responses to repetitive thalamic stimulation, in normal and protein-malnourished adult rats, and found that the rate of cortical incrementation ipsilateral to the thalamic site of stimulation varied as a function of stimulus repetition rate but was largely unaffected by dietary treatment (Figure 7.6). The waveform of the ipsilateral response likewise was unaffected by the protein malnutrition and a characteristic postive-negative response was always observed. On the other hand, in the cortex contralateral to the thalamic stimulation, 7 of 8 protein-

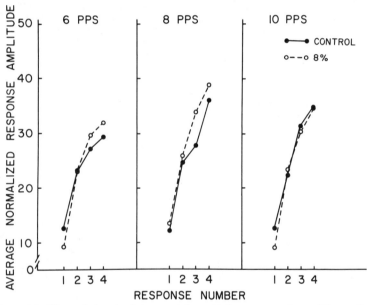

Figure 7.7. Effect of chronic dietary protein restriction on wave-form of the cortical incremental response to thalamic stimulation. Responses are recorded from frontal cortex (Kreig area 10) ipsilateral (I) and contralateral (C) to the stimulated ventral thalamic nucleus in two representative normal protein-reared (NP-2, NP-3) and two low protein-reared (LP-2, LP-4) rats. The normal diet rats were 76 and 77 days of age, while the low-protein rats were 117 and 119 days of age. All traces are averaged responses to the fourth pulse in a 1 sec stimulation train. Pulse repetition rate within trains was 8/sec; surface negativity upward.

102

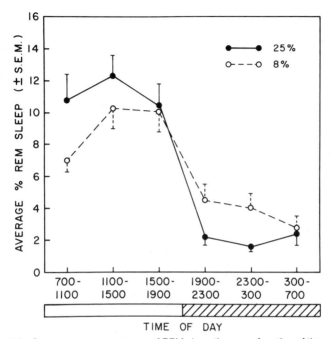

Figure 7.8. Group mean percentages of REM sleep time as a function of time of day. The circadian rhythm (greater amounts of REM during the day, less at night) is less pronounced in the low-protein-fed animals (8 percent) than in the controls (25 percent). This effect was greater in malnourished males than in malnourished females. The fact that the difference between dietary groups is greatest *early* in the light portion and *early* in the dark portion of the day suggests that the effect is associated with changes in the light/dark condition. No such differences between the 8 percent and 25 percent groups were seen with respect to waking or slow-wave sleep.

malnourished animals exhibited a prominent surface negativity (Figure 7.7). These results indicated that the responsiveness of a nonspecific system of the brain was affected even in the adult period by chronic protein malnutrition; the results also support the interpretation that complex central nervous systems, such as the nonspecific, reticularlike assemblies, may be more susceptible to dietary insults than specific sensory pathways such as the visual system.

We would like to summarize our studies of sleep behavior of rats malnourished during development. We found that chronic protein malnutrition did not affect the total relative amounts of waking, slow-wave sleep, and REM in 24 hours. However, this treatment resulted in a reliable shift in the circadian distribution of the REM state (Figure 7.8). Control rats had high levels of REM sleep during the day (700 to 1900 hrs) and low levels during the night (1900 to 700 hrs). Low-protein-fed rats showed a "flatter" circadian distribution of REM sleep. Whereas controls exhibited only about 16 percent of total REM during the night, in low-protein-fed rats nearly 30 percent of total REM occurred during the night. This effect was much more pronounced in males than in females. Further analysis of our data leads us to the tentative conclusion that REM time in the low-protein-fed rats was less affected by changes in the light/dark condition than in controls. We are currently pursuing the possible relationship between these findings and altered endocrine function. Quantitative analysis of the developing sleep states using power spectrum computer techniques are beginning to reveal subtle changes in patterns of electro-ontogenesis, and we are presently carrying out such investigations. In order to better correlate functional development with disturbed anatomy and biochemistry, we plan to pursue studies of electrogenesis wherever the biochemical, anatomical, or behavioral studies provide leads.

Ontogenetic Development of Biogenic Amines in Brain and Peripheral Tissues in Protein-malnourished Rats

During the past two decades increasing attention has been given to the effects of protein or protein-calorie malnutrition on the development of the central nervous system. As is well known, malnutrition during early development has been found to affect many aspects of the maturation of the brain in the offspring. However, in most experimental studies the malnutrition regimen has been initiated during the postnatal period of development, thus preventing an evaluation of the effects of prenatal malnutrition. Also, the majority of investigators have employed the technique of either increasing the number of offspring per dam or reducing access to the lactating mother. These factors cause alterations in the social environment during rearing, making it difficult to evaluate which changes in central nervous-system functioning are caused by inadequate nutrition and which by "rearing variables" or the interaction between these two factors. In our studies we investigated the effects of rearing rats on a diet low in protein, introduced prior to mating, on the ontogeny of monoamines and 5-hydroxyindoleacetic acid levels in regional brain areas. To assess the specificity of amine changes observed in the brain, serotonin, norepinephrine, and 5-hydroxyindoleacetic acid concentrations were also measured in peripheral tissues.

We examined the ontogeny of the biogenic amines in protein-malnourished rats because: (a) these amines have been shown to play key roles in many aspects of behavior; and (b) they are synthesized from amino acid precursors and are usually affected by deficiencies in dietary protein. By determining the nature of the effects of early protein malnutrition on brain serotonin and norepinephrine systems we sought to increase our understanding of the biochemical bases of the electrophysiological and behavioral disturbances which we have described in such subjects. In order to parallel many human malnutrition conditions, we initiated the low protein (8 percent casein) diet prior to pregnancy and continued it through gestation, lactation, and for long periods after weaning. Measurements of serotonin, 5-hydroxyindoleacetic acid, and norepinephrine were made from birth to age 300 days.

At most ages brains of the 8 percent casein animals had significantly higher serotonin, 5-hydroxyindoleacetic acid, and norepinephrine levels than the normal control groups (Figures 7.9 and 7.10).[26] The regional brain analyses showed that these neurochemicals were, as expected, more highly concentrated in subtelencephalic brain regions, that is, in the diencephalon, midbrain, and pons-medulla regions (Figure 7.11). The region-dependent nature of the diet effects were most pronounced at ages 0, 21, 60, 145, and 300 days with significant increases in levels in the 8 percent rats ranging from 30 to 200 percent or more.

Analyses of amine and 5-hydroxyindoleacetic acid levels in peripheral tissues also showed marked diet-related effects. Serotonin and/or 5-hydroxyindoleacetic acid concentrations in lung, heart, and stomach were significantly higher at most age points in the 8 percent groups than in the controls, the average increase being about 30 to 200 percent. Norepinephrine levels, however, were not markedly altered at any ages examined in the 8 percent rats.

The results of these studies indicated that developmental protein malnutrition elevated brain and peripheral tissue concentrations of serotonin and 5-hydroxyindoleacetic acid at most ages even though the low-protein diet was deficient in the amino acid

105

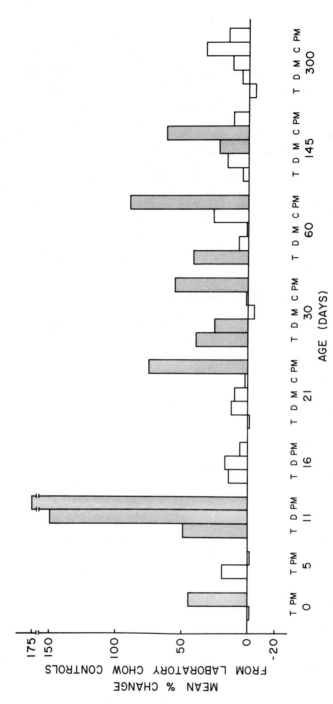

Figure 7.9. Ontogenetic effects of a chronic low-protein (8 percent casein) diet on regional brain serotonin levels. Abbreviations: T = telencephalon; PM = pons-medulla; D = diencephalon; M = midbrain; C = cerebellum. Darkened bars indicate statistically significant differences in percent change compared to laboratory chow controls. For further details, see tables of chemistry data in Stern et al.[26]

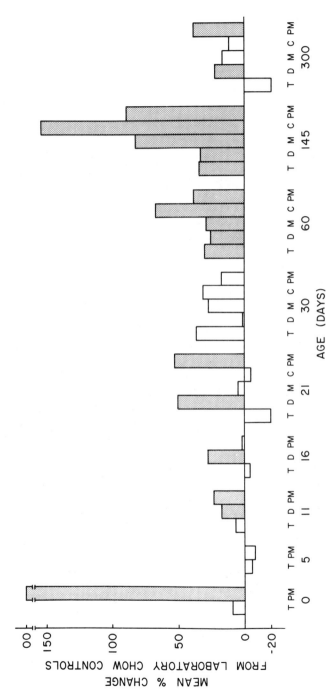

Figure 7.10. Ontogenetic effects of a chronic low-protein (8 percent casein) diet on regional brain norepinephrine levels. Abbreviations: T = telencephalon; PM = pons-medulla; D = diencephalon; M = midbrain; C = cerebellum. Darkened bars indicate statistically significant differences in percent change compared to laboratory chow controls For further details see tables of chemistry data in Stern et al.[26]

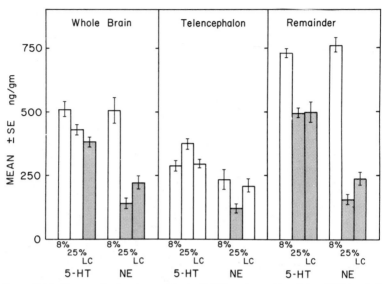

Figure 7.11. Bar graph showing serotonin (5-HT) and norepinephrine (NE) levels in whole brain, telencephalon, and remainder of brain on day of birth. Stippled bars indicate significant differences from the 8 percent casein group. "Remainder" in this figure refers primarily to the brainstem values. Abbreviations: 8 percent = 8 percent casein diet; 25 percent = 25 percent casein diet; LC = laboratory chow diet.

precursor of the indoles, that is, tryptophan. The regional brain distribution of the increases in indole levels in the malnourished rats indicated that the telencephalon was least affected, while most of the increase occurred in the brainstem (Figure 7.11). Since the midbrain and pons-medulla contain the serotonin perikarya of the central nervous system, it would appear that the effects of protein malnutrition were most clearly manifested at the level of the areas containing the cell bodies.

The increases in serotonin and 5-hydroxyindoleacetic acid concentrations in peripheral tissues of the 8 percent animals suggest that indole changes represented a general alteration in serotonin metabolism and that the brain was not necessarily "spared" from neurochemical changes seen in peripheral organs of malnourished rats. The reason for the increase in serotonin and metabolite concentrations was not clear so that further study of indole metabolism, especially tryptophan availability in the malnourished condition, is now underway in our laboratory.

Regional brain norepinephrine concentration analyses showed

that at most ages the malnourished rats had significantly greater levels than the control groups. with the largest increases occurring in the midbrain and pons-medulla areas. This again suggests that the effect of protein malnutrition was localized to the cell bodies of the noradrenergic neurons in the midbrain and pons-medulla regions and not at the forebrain noradrenergic terminal areas. In contrast to serotonin, no changes were found in peripheral tissue concentrations of norepinephrine in the 8 percent rats at any age examined. This suggests that, in the case of norepinephrine, the brain was more sensitive to the insult of protein malnutrition than were peripheral tissues.

Perhaps one of the most important aspects of our biochemical studies is that large changes in the biogenic amine content of the brain were observed within 24 hours after birth, well before the start of one well-defined brain-growth spurt period in the rat (Figure 7.12). The brain-growth spurt period has been widely considered to be the ontogenetic intervals when malnutrition would most likely exert the most debilitating effects on the central ner-

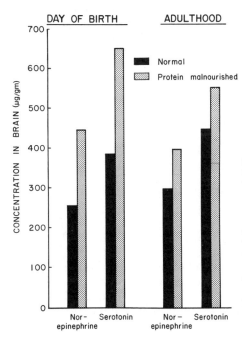

Figure 7.12. Bar graph comparing norepinephrine and serotonin values in normal (black bars) and protein-malnourished (stippled bars) rats on day of birth and at adulthood. The values on the ordinate are nanograms/gram from whole brain determinations. The normal diets in this instance was laboratory chow. Adults are 60-day-old rats. Day of birth values are means of 12 brain determinations. Adult values are means of 6 brain determinations. See also Stern et al.[26]

109

P. J. Morgane et al.

vous system.[7] However, the changes observed in 0 to 24-hour-old neonate brain amines demonstrated that, in the rat, maternal protein restriction begun prior to gestation could markedly alter the neurochemical profile of the brains of the offspring. What significance the changes in biogenic amine and 5-hydroxyindoleacetic acid levels have for the later behavioral capabilities of the protein-malnourished rats remains to be evaluated. The fundamental role(s) which serotonin and norepinephrine play in learning, memory, sleep, aggression, reaction to stress, and so on, suggest that disturbances might occur in all these aspects of behavior of rats that are protein malnourished during development.

In analyzing the chemistry data, several points need to be emphasized. The concept of the brain growth spurt and vulnerable period has been discussed by Dobbing and his group. This concept states that the brain is most vulnerable to insults during periods of brain growth spurt. In addition, the possibility exists that the adverse effects on the brain may be partially or completely reversed by suitable treatment during the brain growth spurt. In our studies, the protein-malnourished rats (8 percent casein) showed elevated brain levels of serotonin and norepinephrine from birth to age 300 days. Since the brain growth spurt in rats is almost entirely postnatal, we have demonstrated a major biochemical change in the brains of neonates whose mothers were protein restricted *before* the brain growth spurt. If these data can be extrapolated to humans, all three trimesters of pregnancy become important with respect to vulnerability of the developing brain in utero.

The elevated brain levels of serotonin and norepinephrine in the 0 to 24-hour-old experimental neonates become even more significant when one considers that the brain weights of the experimental and control neonates were essentially similar. It is important to emphasize here that the diets used in our studies were isocaloric. The experimental diet contained less protein (8 percent casein) than the control diet (25 percent casein) and contained additional carbohydrate to make up for the decrease in calories due to the reduction in protein content. Our studies indicated that during gestation the mothers fed the 8 percent casein diet actually ate more per gram body weight than did the mothers fed the control diet. Since the diets were isocaloric, the protein-restricted mothers did not suffer caloric restriction and, in fact, may have had an increased caloric intake. Thus, the biochemical

110

changes seen in the experimental rat at birth seemed to be the result of protein restriction of the mother in the presence of an abundance of calories in the diet during gestation. Determination of the influence that protein-calorie or calorie restriction has on the developing nervous system during gestation and lactation requires suitable controlled studies. We are currently investigating the mechanisms which may possibly be responsible for the elevated brain levels of serotonin and norepinephrine in the protein-deprived animals. We studied the synthesis rate of brain serotonin in adult rats reared on the 8 percent and 25 percent casein diets using monoamine oxidase inhibition by pargyline. The results showed that serotonin synthesis was comparable in the two groups. We also determined that reserpine administration resulted in a depletion of serotonin and norepinephrine in both groups of animals, with a concomitant increase in 5-hydroxyindoleacetic acid. Thus, it would seem that the synthesis rates and the degradative rates for brain serotonin were comparable in both groups of animals. This was further corroborated by the fact that we found comparable levels of the monoamine oxidase (MAO) enzyme system in isolated synaptosomes obtained from both groups of animals.

We are currently investigating the possibility that the protein-deprived animals have higher brain levels of serotonin and norepinephrine as a consequence of higher levels of precursor amino acids in the brain. Preliminary data indicated that the levels of free tryptophan in the brains of the experimental animals were markedly greater than in the controls. This would seem to be a remarkable adaption by the organism to a relative decreased amount of protein both in the diet and in the circulation. Additional preliminary data indicated that growth hormone and possibly adrenal corticoids may have been involved in this adaptation to protein restriction in the diet. Since we observed a decreased ATPase activity in isolated synaptosomes obtained from the protein-deprived rats (see below) and, since amines are stored in vesicles bound to ATP, a decreased ATPase activity could possibly result in an increased store of the biogenic amines.

Recovery of Synaptosomal Na +/K + ATPase in Post-weaned Protein-deficient Rats

A large body of evidence cites the impairment of neuronal development resulting from prenatal and postnatal protein malnutrition. The synaptosomes, which are broken fragments of nerve-ending structures recovered by centrifugal techniques, provide a basis for specific study of a limited number of important neuronal biochemical functions. One of these functions, Na+/K+ ATPase activity, plays an important role in maintaining the ionic gradients essential for nerve-impulse conduction.

The specific activity of Na+/K+ stimulated ATPase developed progressively in synaptosomal fractions of the cerebrum and cerebellum over the 21-day postnatal period. Subsequently the specific activity progressively decreased to 42 days of life, and at 63 days remained equivalent to the 42-day value (Figures 7.13 and 7.14). The development of this enzyme in those neonates maintained on low-protein diets (10 percent casein) during gestation and lactation was significantly impaired as reflected by the lower specific activities of this enzyme in synaptosomal fractions derived from the two brain regions at 14 days and 21 days of life. The cerebellar development at and after 42 days of age differed

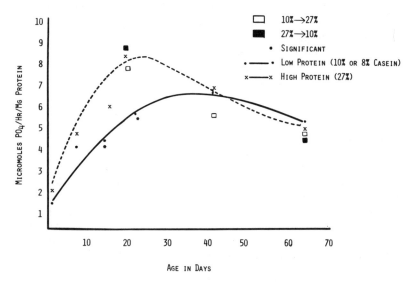

Figure 7.13. Effect of protein-deficient diet (10 percent casein) fed during the gestation period on neonatal cerebellar synaptosomal Na +/K + ATPase activity. Diet maintained through 63 days of age. Diet switching (10%⇌27%) instituted at birth, 21 and 42 days of age, continuing for a 21-day period. Data listed in Table 7.1.

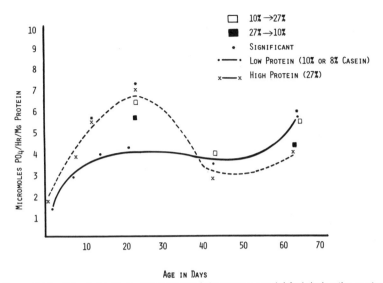

AGE IN DAYS

Figure 7.14. Effect of protein-deficient diet (10 percent casein) fed during the gestation period on neonatal cerebral synaptosomal Na + /K + ATPase activity. Diet maintained through 63 days of age. Diet switching (10%⇌27%) instituted at birth, 21 and 42 days of age, continuing for a 21-day period. Data listed in Table 7.1.

from the cerebrum. In the cerebellum the $Na+/K+$ ATPase activity was equivalent for the low-protein and control groups at 42 and 63 days of age. In the cerebrum at 63 days of age, the specific activity in the low-protein group was significantly ($p > 0.004$) increased over the control group (Table 7.1). Cerebellar activity would suggest that protein insufficiency delayed development, but that ultimately normal $Na+/K+$ ATPase activity levels were reached.

The effect of gestational protein insufficiency upon $Na+/K+$ ATPase appeared to be reversible at birth by augmenting the diet with protein (27 percent casein). Equally important is the fact that protein insufficiency imposed upon gestationally well-nourished neonates at the time of birth did not diminish the specific $Na+/K+$ ATPase activity in the cerebellar synaptosomes; however, the activity was reduced in the cerebrum under the same conditions.

In view of the apparent regional difference in susceptibility to malnutrition during the lactation period, synaptic development

Table 7.1. Effect of protein diet on Na+/K+ mg stimulated ATPase activity in rat brain synaptosomes. Values stated in columns 6, 7, and 8 are for whole brain preparation.

Age (D)	Diet	N	Cerebellum	P*	N	Cerebrum	P*
1	10%	(8)	1.273 ± .113	.04			
	27%	(7)	2.057 ± .901				
7	10%	(4)	3.881 ± 1.179	.51	(5)	2.944 ± 1.104	.23
	27%	(5)	4.683 ± 2.360		(5)	3.974 ± 1.374	
14	10%	(6)	4.202 ± .616	.031	(6)	3.817 ± 1.104	.021
	27%	(6)	5.744 ± 1.354		(7)	5.606 ± 1.319	
21	10%	(5)	5.422 ± .704	.0001	(5)	4.188 ± 1.639	.019
	27%	(8)	8.157 ± .949		(7)	6.700 ± 1.353	
21 Reversal at birth	10%–27%	(16)	7.736 ± 1.368	.38	(16)	6.701 ± 1.305	.56
	27%–10%	(5)	8.327 ± 1.449	.56	(5)	5.769 ± 2.160	.39
42	10%	(6)	6.342 ± 1.587	.56	(5)	3.462 ± 1.423	.44
	27%	(7)	6.475 ± 1.113		(7)	2.893 ± .660	
42 Reversal at 21 days	8%–25%	(9)	5.296 ± 1.060	.06	(9)	3.774 ± .941	.054
63	8%	(4)	5.032 ± 1.000	.57	(4)	5.599 ± 1.216	.004
	25%	(4)	4.860 ± .510		(4)	3.854 ± .695	
63 Reversal at 42 days	10%–27%	(6)	4.772 ± 1.710	.56	(6)	5.443 ± 1.216	.032
	27%–10%	(10)	4.574 ± 1.105	.50	(8)	3.998 ± 1.197	.56

*P values derived from the comparison to the high-protein dietary group at each age category.

may occur at different rates. To determine the plasticity of the synaptosome development relative to membranous Na+/K+ AT-Pase activity as a function of neonatal age, diet reversal studies were conducted. Diets were reversed (27 percent casein to 10 percent casein, or 10 percent to 27 percent) after weaning (21 days) and 42 days of age, and in each case continued for an additional 21 days (data summarized in Table 7.1). These data indicated that irrespective of the diet (10 percent or 27 percent fed during the lactation and postweanling period) levels of synaptosomal Na+/K+ ATPase activities at 42 days of age were equivalent within each brain region. Further, protein diet augmentation at 21 days of age did not alter the ATPase activities ultimately reached at 42 days of age. Neonates which were maintained on either a high- or low-protein diet for 42 days followed by diet reversal for 21 days, until an age of 63 days, had normal levels of synaptosomal Na+/K+ ATPase activity in the cerebellum. The specific activity for the cerebrum, however, was increased and equivalent to the low-protein group at this age (10 to 27 percent).

Feeding augmented protein diets (27 percent) at birth increased to normal levels the synaptosomal Na+/K+ ATPase activity by 21 days of age. However, maintaining the animals for an extended period of 42 days on the 10 percent casein diet produced an equivalent level of enzyme activity as the 27 percent casein control group. These data would suggest that the primary effect of low-protein diet administered during gestation was to delay development. Ultimately, normal levels of enzyme activity were reached. Early dietary intervention accelerated "catch-up" development. Postweanling protein dietary intervention had little effect on the synaptosomal Na+/K+ ATPase activity in either brain region. However, the cerebral activity at 63 days of age was significantly increased in the low-protein (10 percent) group and was not altered by diet augmentation at 42 days of age. These data suggested a regional difference in response to low-protein diet.

Behavioral Effects of Chronic Protein Malnutrition: Acquisition and Long-term Retention of a Temporal Discrimination

One of the more important issues concerning the effects of chronic exposure to low-protein diets during development and adulthood is the question of whether this dietary regimen produces subjects with learning and/or memory deficits. A behavioral test situation that is well suited for evaluating this question in the rat is an alternation (go/no-go) discrimination. In this task the subject must correctly recall the outcome of the prior trial in order to correctly respond on the next trial.[13] The present set of three studies employed a discrete trial procedure in which the stimuli signalling the onset of the reinforced trial (S$^+$) or the nonreinforced trial (S$^-$) were the same, that is, the onset of a house light. Lever presses were followed by water reinforcement only on alternate trials—responding on the S$^-$ trials was not punished, but no reinforcement was delivered and such responses were scored as errors. The measure of the level of discrimination performance was the ratio between the number of S⁻ trials responsed to, divided by the number of correct S⁺ trials. A ratio of 1.00 indicated a failure to discriminate S⁻ from S⁺ trials; a ratio of 0.5 indicated a fairly good level of discrimination.

There were several advantages to using the single-alternation paradigm for evaluating the rate of acquisition performance and long-term memory status in protein-malnourished rats. First, this task involved a strong short-term memory component, since correct performance required recall of the prior trial. By manipulating the interval between the S⁻ and S⁺ trials it was possible to assess whether the performance of protein-malnourished rats was impaired on tasks requiring a greater utilization of short-term memory. Secondly, the temporal aspect of this alternation, as opposed to spatial alternation, reduced the possibility of the formation of positioning responses as a means for mediating the discrimination. Also, the present alternation task did not employ shock or other markedly aversive stimuli. This was important since we and others have found that protein-malnourished rats have heightened physiological[27] and behavioral[16] reactivity to noxious events.

The first study examined the acquisition rates of adult normal rats (25 percent casein diet) and protein-malnourished rats (8 percent casein diet) on a single alternation discrimination with trial duration of 12 sec and an intertrial interval (ITI) of 8 sec.[25] The discrimination ratio results (Figure 7.15) showed that the malnourished rats acquired this discrimination to a significantly poorer extent than the normals. However, the acquisition curves in Figure 7.15 are essentially parallel, indicating that learning, once it began, occurred at the same rate in both normal and malnourished rats. This observation that the learning rates over session blocks ##2 to 7 were highly similar in the normal and malnourished rats suggests that the initial delay in acquisition within block #1 in the malnourished rats was not due to a learning deficit, but was rather a performance impairment.

A second study employing subjects from the prior experiment determined whether training on a more difficult alternation discrimination would produce differences in learning rates between normal and protein-malnourished rats. In this study an 18 sec ITI was employed, compared to an 8 sec ITI in the prior study. The results of this experiment, shown in Figure 7.16, were quite similar to that of the prior 8 sec ITI study. Although there were signifi-

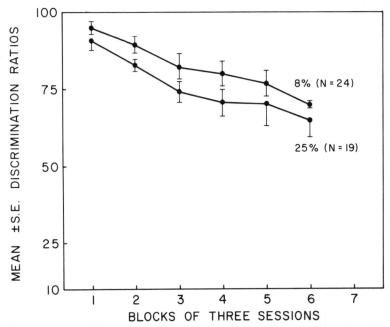

Figure 7.15. Acquisition performance of normal (25 percent casein) and protein-malnourished (8 percent casein) rats on an alternation discrimination test in which lever presses were followed by water reward only on alternate trials. An intertrial-interval (ITI) of 8 sec was employed. The discrimination ratio on the ordinate is the number of nonreinforced trials responded to, divided by the number of reinforced trials responded to × 100. A ratio of 100 represents equal responding on both types of trials, that is, failure of the alternation discrimination. An anlysis of variance indicated significantly poorer performance by the malnourished rats.

cant differences between the normal and malnourished discrimination ratios, the acquisition curves were parallel, thus indicating comparable acquisition rates after the initial block of 3 sessions.

The third study employed a subset of subjects from the first two studies, which were matched for equal performance and tested on (a) the long-term retention of the alternation discrimination, and (b) the reacquisition rates of the 18 sec ITI discrimination. In the long-term retention test 30 days elapsed between the end of session block #7 of study #2 (18 sec ITI) and the retention test on the 18 sec ITI task in study #3. The results, shown in Figure 7.17 (dashed lines) indicated a comparable degree of forgetting in the

P. J. Morgane et al.

normal and protein-malnourished rats. In both groups the discrimination ratios deteriorated from about 40 at the end of study #2 to about 75 at the start of the retention test in study #3.

The results of the retraining sessions in this study (Figure 7.17) showed a significantly faster relearning rate by the normal rats than by the malnourished subjects. In this case the performance curves for the two groups sharply separated between session blocks #2 and #3. This suggests there was a difference in learning rates rather than a performance impairment as found in the prior two studies. Faster acquisition rates by normal rats in this test situation support the view that tasks in which learning is heavily based upon utilization of previously acquired long-term memories are less readily acquired by chronically protein-malnourished rats. Further exploration of this concept using a latent-learning paradigm should reveal whether chronic devel-

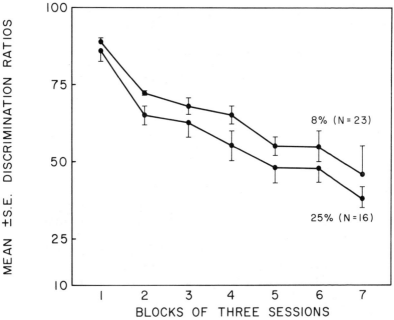

Figure 7.16. Acquisition performance on an alternation discrimination with an intertrial-interval (ITI) of 18 sec by normal and protein-malnourished rats. The malnourished rats performed at a significantly poorer level than the normal rats.

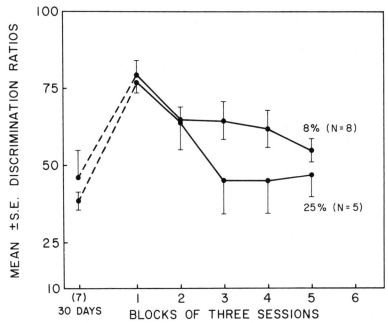

Figure 7.17. Long-term retention and relearning of an alternation discrimination employing an intertrial-interval (ITI) of 18 sec by normal and protein-malnourished rats. The dashed lines represent the 30-day interval between completion of training block #7 of Figure 7.16 and the retention test on block #1. Significant differences occurred in the relearning rates between the normal and malnourished rats.

opmental protein malnutrition leads to a generalized impairment in the ability to integrate complex long-term memories in the development of ongoing discrimination behavior.

Morphological Studies of the Effects of Protein Malnutrition on the Developing Brain

In our recent morphological studies we showed that only by the parameter of the ratio of brain weight to body weight did rats raised on a low-protein diet resemble controls of a younger age. In these protein-restricted rats the proportion of the brain which is neocortex, archicortex, and cerebellum was the same as in controls. Camera lucida drawings of rapid Golgi-impregnated neurons of these undernourished rats resembled age-matched controls. Only in quantitative studies of rapid Golgi-impregnated

119

neurons did differences between the two groups appear. These differences included significant reduction in dendritic length of neurons in the cortex and cerebellum and a decrease in spine density in the neocortex and cerebellum in malnourished rats at 30 days of age. Although the complete significance of these findings is not known, they did show that undernutrition had a clearcut morphological effect on the developing brain. Current investigations by our group are now focusing on similar quantitative Golgi studies of subcortical formations of the brain. These include investigations of a nucleate neuronal assembly, that is, the striatum, and a reticulate neuronal assembly, that is, the diagonal band of Broca. Analysis of these formations, which are simpler in their organization than the cortical (laminate) structures, may shed light on the morphological derangements produced by protein malnutrition by providing a more detailed picture of abnormal neuronal differentiation and connectivity.

References

1. Astic, L., and D. Jouvet-Mounier. Etude polygraphique et comportémentale des états de vigilance chez le cobaye prématuré. *Physiol. Behav.* 7: 59–64, 1971.
2. Boyer, S., and G. R. Kirk. Maturation of the visual evoked response in the dog. *Exp. Neurol.* 38: 449–457, 1973.
3. Bronzino, J., P. J. Morgane, W. B. Forbes, W. C. Stern, and O. Resnick. Ontogeny of visual evoked responses in rats protein-deprived during development. *Biol. Psychiat.* 10: 175–184, 1975.
4. Callison, D. A., and J. W. Spencer. Effect of chronic undernutrition and/or visual deprivation upon the visual evoked potential from the developing rat brain. *Devel. Psychobiol.* 1: 196–204, 1968.
5. Crain, S. M. Development of electrical activity in the cerebral cortex of the albino rat. *Proc. Soc. Exp. Biol. Med.* 81: 49–51, 1952.
6. Dahlstrom, A., and K. Fuxe. Evidence for the existence of monoamine-containing neurons in the central nervous system. *Acta Physiol. Scand.* Suppl. 232, 62: 1–55, 1964.
7. Dobbing, J. Effects of experimental undernutrition on development of the nervous system. In *Malnutrition, Learning, and Behavior*, N. S. Scrimshaw and J. E. Gordon, eds., M.I.T. Press, Cambridge, Mass., 1968, pp. 181–202.
8. Ellingson, R. J. Development of wakefulness-sleep cycles and associated EEG patterns in mammals. In *Sleep and the Maturing Nervous System*, C. D. Clemente, D. P. Purpura, and F. E. Mayer, eds., Academic Press, New York, 1972, pp. 165–174.

9. Ellingson, R. J., and G. H. Rose. Ontogenesis of the electroencephalogram. In *Developmental Neurobiology*, W. Himwich, ed., Charles C. Thomas, Springfield, Springfield, Ill., 1970, pp. 441–474.

10. Engel, R. Abnormal brain wave patterns in kwashiorkor. *EEG Clin. Neurophysiol.* 8: 489–500, 1956.

11. Forbes, William B., Oscar Resnick, Warren C. Stern, Joseph D. Bronzino, Peter J. Morgane, The effect of chronic protein malnutrition on trans-callosal evoked responses in the rat. *Devel. Psychobiol.* 8: 503–509, 1975.

12. Gramsbergen, A. Neuro-ontogeny of sleep in the rat. In *Basic Sleep Mechanisms*, O. Petre-Quadens and J. D. Schlag, eds., Academic Press, New York, 1974, pp. 339–353.

13. Heise, G. A. Discrete trial analysis of drug action. *Fed. Proc.* 34: 1898–1903, 1975.

14. Huttenlocher, P. R. Development of cortical neuronal activity in the neonatal cat. *Exp. Neurol.* 17: 247–262, 1967.

15. Jouvet-Mounier, D., L. Astic, and D. Lacote. Ontogenesis of the states of sleep in rat, cat, and guinea pig during the first postnatal month. *Devel. Psychobiol.* 2: 216–239, 1970.

16. Levitsky, D. A., and R. H. Barnes. Effect of early malnutrition on the reaction of adult rats to aversive stimuli. *Nature* 225: 468–469, 1970.

17. MacFadyen, U. M., I. Oswald, and S. A. Lewis. Starvation and human slow-wave sleep. *J. Appl. Physiol.* 35: 391–394, 1973.

18. Mares, P., and Z. Vitova. Visual evoked cortical potentials in adult rats. *Physiologia Bohemoslovaca* 21: 623–628, 1972.

19. Nelson, G. K. The electroencephalogram in kwashiorkor. *EEG Clin. Neurophysiol.* 11: 73–84, 1959.

20. Parmelee, A. H., W. H. Wenner, Y. Akiyama, E. Stern, and J. Flescher. Electroencephalography and brain maturation. In *Regional Development of the Brain in Early Life*, A. Minkowski, ed., Oxford, Blackwell Scientific Publications, 1967, pp. 459–476.

21. Rose, G. H. The development of visually evoked electrocortical responses in the rat. *Devel. Psychobiol.* 1: 35–40, 1968.

22. Rosen, M. G., and A. McLaughlin. Fetal and maternal electroencephalography in the guinea pig. *Exp. Neurol.* 16: 181–190, 1966.

23. Salas, M., and L. Cintra. Nutritional influences upon somatosensory evoked responses during development in the rat. *Physiol. Behav.* 10: 1019–1022, 1973.

24. Seggie, J., and M. Berry. Ontogeny of interhemispheric evoked potentials in the rat: Significance of myelination of the corpus callosum. *Exp. Neurol.* 35: 215–232, 1972.

25. Stern, W. C., W. B. Forbes, O. Resnick, and P. J. Morgane. Seizure susceptibility and brain amine levels following protein malnutrition during development in the rat. *Brain Res.* 79: 375–384, 1974.

26. Stern, W. C., M. Miller, W. B. Forbes, P. J. Morgane, and O. Resnick. Ontogeny of the levels of biogenic amines in various parts of the brain and in peripheral tissues in normal and protein malnourished rats. *Exp. Neurol.* 49: 314–326, 1975a.

27. Stern, W. C., P. J. Morgane, M. Miller, and O. Resnick. Protein malnutrition in rats: Response of brain amines and behavior to foot shock stress. *Exp. Neurol.* 47: 56–67, 1975b.

28. Tuge, H., Y. Kanayama, and C. H. Yueh. Comparative studies on the development of EEG. *Japan. J. Physiol.* 10: 211–220, 1960.

Seymour Levine **8**

Discussion

In the early 1900's a raging controversy centered around Cornell concerning two fundamental schools of thought called structuralism and functionalism. It is rather interesting that today we find ourselves right back at the same place. What we have in the preceding chapters and in the field of malnutrition and behavior shows an enormous discrepancy between structuralist and functionalist positions. We have individuals who look at structure and developing systems, and we have individuals who look at functions, and somehow they do not quite seem to be relevant to each other. For example, let me cite from Zamenhof's paper.[1] Zamenhof said that he observed a significant difference in learning ability in animals of the F_2 generation. There is an essential fallacy in that statement. If we look closely at the *Developmental Psychobiology* paper from which this is quoted, we will find a learning deficiency only in the ninth and tenth reversal task. If we look at original learning and several reversal learnings thereafter, we find there is no deficiency whatsoever; so if there is a deficiency in learning, it is very subtle.

I have been in the animal business for 25 years. In that period I have wiped out my animal colony three times because of illness. Yet in the literature on malnutrition and behavior we find large groups of people making inferences about animals that are tested while sick: animals that are examined while malnourished *are* sick and lethargic and obviously have behavioral deficits, and to make inferences about brain function from animals that are tested when in a very poor state, animals that are in some instances at 60 to 70 percent of their body weight, is erroneous.

Let us return to this functional and structural proposition. Zamenhof speaks of his malnourished animals as damaged and impaired. Yet I believe that if I were to look at the literature, I should ask, in what way are malnourished animals damaged? I am

123

saying exactly what John Dobbing said in his paper: In what way are they functionally impaired? If we go through the literature in detail, in terms of nutritionally rehabilitated animals, we find that recovery is much more the rule than the exception. Let us take, for example, the study that was presented by Fernstrom and Lytle (see Chapter 6 above). Yes, deficiencies are there, depending upon which aspect of the data is emphasized. They chose to emphasize changes that occurred during the period of malnutrition, yet they observed complete recovery when they reinstated the animals' normal diet. If we review the literature extensively, we find there are very few real instances of permanent behavioral impairment.

It is perhaps notable that one of the groups that finds replicable differences is the Cornell group. Their methods, however, are different from anybody else's. They use seven weeks of postnatal malnutrition, not three weeks of preweaning malnutrition. If the critical period for brain changes occurs during the preweaning period, why are the additional four weeks of postweaning malnutrition needed to show behavioral impairment? In addition, the impairment of behavior after seven weeks of malnutrition is found only in males. It doesn't occur in females. These findings are buried in their literature and not brought out extensively. Thus, the behavioral differences observed after seven weeks of postnatal malnutrition cannot be generalized to both sexes.

A rather interesting set of dichotomies exists between the structuralists and the functionalists. The structuralist would like to believe that structural changes are those which produce damage, and yet for those of us who have been involved in development for a very long time, the one thing with which we are very impressed is not the vulnerability but the plasticity of the system. Developmental systems are inordinately plastic, and there is a whole realm of evidence on the plasticity of the nervous system and its ability to adjust. Yet we still tend to emphasize vulnerability rather than resiliency. What I want to point out is that "damage(s)" and "impairment" during the period of malnutrition do not necessarily represent irreversible changes in function. At many later points in development, regardless of what the hardware (brain) changes may be, there seems to be little evidence that the hardware changes are related to behavior.

In addition, I would like to present some data we have collected that challenges yet another proposition: that while an organism is malnourished, it is retarded in development. There is much evidence that psychomotor and behavioral development is retarded during the preweaning period as the result of early malnutrition. Sandra Wiener and I have recently completed a series of studies looking at the maturation of the pituitary-adrenal system of the perinatally malnourished rat. We found an acceleration of development, not retardation. We found an organism that presumably had all these "damaged" structural changes, and yet in one system, the organism had not been at all retarded. Figure 8.1 shows the differences. The rat normally does not show a pituitary-adrenal response to stress at 10 days of age. It does not begin to respond until somewhere between 15 and 16 days of age. However, the animals we tested (malnourished by giving the mother an 8 percent protein diet) clearly showed a marked basal elevation and very active response to stress at 14 days of age as compared with controls—which did not yet show a stress response at that age. The system was therefore not retarded; rather it appears to be accelerated.

Another rather interesting indication is that the basal corticosteroid level is higher. At day 18 and day 22, when both control and malnourished animals were responding to stress, elevation of

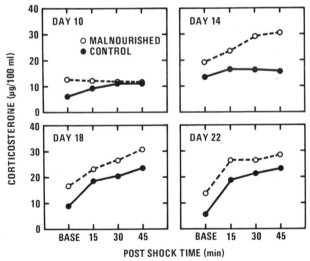

Figure 8.1. Plasma corticosterone concentration as a function of postshock interval, malnutrition, and age

basal levels continued in the malnourished pups. One might say that the basal level was higher because these animals were "stressed" due to malnutrition, but it is not as simple as this. The animals in Figure 8.1 were picked up and weighed every other day in order to generate a growth curve. Figure 8.2 shows the basal corticoid level of malnourished and control rats, some of which were handled and some not. In handled malnourished litters there was an elevation of basal levels. No rise was observed in the nonhandled malnourished litters. Thus, the elevated basal level was not due to malnutrition alone but was a consequence of the handling interacting with the malnutrition and presumably altering the mother and infant relationship.

Yet, given all of these differences, when we observed these animals as adults after nutritional rehabilitation begun at weaning was completed, we could not find any difference in corticosteroid levels due to early malnutrition. Figure 8.3 shows the results of four or five different kinds of stress situations. The only difference that is apparent is a sex difference. There is no effect of the early malnutrition. One might say that we did not use the appropriate time parameter. Figure 8.4 shows the results of a time course. We observed no functional pituitary-adrenal response difference in any of these systems as a consequence of early malnutrition.

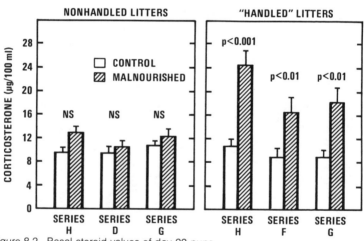

Figure 8.2. Basal steroid values of day 22 pups

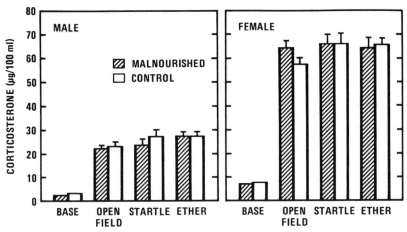

Figure 8.3. Adult steroid data

Unfortunately, sides are going to be taken here, and the sides are very clearly demarcated. On the one hand is the position John Dobbing takes, which, given my bias, I must cheer:

> To the uninitiated the research strategy which has been employed over the years in the study of our subject must seem misguided, to say the least. The logical progression would have been first to look for lasting effects of early growth restriction on behaviour and then, if any were found, to seek correlated changes in the brain. If anything, the reverse order has been followed. The flow of information on vulnerability of brain structure has largely preceded that on vulnerability of behaviour. The principal reason for this state of affairs is the relative ease with which the grosser aspects of brain morphology and composition can be measured, coupled with the immaturity and imprecision of the behavioural sciences. Now the indisputable evidence is that early growth restriction results in both deficits and distortions in brain growth, and the burden is on the behaviourist to determine whether or not this matters.[2]

This point is very clearly the case. The fact that you see changes in growth, that you see changes in DNA and RNA, that you see changes in cell number, that you see changes in dendritic growth, are all indisputable. Whether or not this matters, I think is the major question.

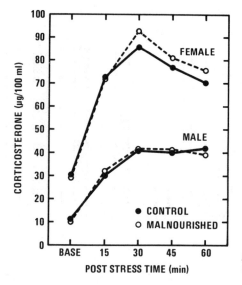

Figure 8.4. Adult steroid time course

References

1. Bressler, D., G. Ellison, and S. Zamenhof. Learning deficits in rats with malnourished grandmothers. *Developmental Psychobiol.* 8: 315, 1975.

2. Dobbing, J., and J. Smart. Vulnerability of developing brain and behavior. *Brit. Med. Bull.* 30: 165, 1974.

Discussion

We have here two major kinds of disagreement. One is illustrated by the differences between Stephen Zamenhof and John Dobbing and represents a controversy *within* the area. The other disagreement is illustrated by Seymour Levine and is directed *at* the area. Let us consider in detail where the agreements and disagreements stand.

I think it is fair to say, concerning the Dobbing-Zamenhof controversy, that there are some very substantial agreements. Basically, they agree in terms of the data; this is really very important. Where they disagree is in the interpretation of the data. They both agree that brain biochemistry can be altered during prenatal development of the rat. They agree that this can happen early in development and that the effects of malnutrition during gestation on the brain chemistry in humans is largely unknown. They also agree that there are two pieces of data in the literature which have to be explained in the context of their interpretations. Data from the Susser and Stein study showed that severe prenatal nutrition alone in a nondeprived population had very few if any effects on later performance. On the other hand, the accumulating data from a number of developing countries demonstrates that severe prenatal malnutrition alone in a deprived population does affect performance, independent of the postnatal nutritional state.

Where do they disagree? Dobbing says that the human brain is protected during the critical period—which occurs earlier in humans than in the rat and at a time when the brain is protected against malnutrition. He notes there is no evidence of any effect of malnutrition on the human brain during this period. Moreover, he believes that the recovery period postnatally and during the late portion of pregnancy is long enough in the development of the human brain to allow recovery even if certain subtle changes occur.

Zamenhof, on the other hand, says that the human brain may not be protected prenatally. He cites as evidence the fact that early malnutrition may affect the physiology and the biochemistry of the mother and the placenta, leading to changes quite apart from the concurrent nutritional changes as they occur on the fetus. He cites as supporting evidence that, in the rat, long-term biochemical changes in the brain can be demonstrated even if the malnutrition is present only for the first or second day of gestation. He has no data, of course, in terms of the human.

Lastly, Zamenhof takes the position that there may be events that can occur only early in development; and recovery of an insult at that time may never be rehabilitatable.

It is tougher to deal with Levine's criticisms. Levine is concerned with the claims of long-term behavioral effects. He states that recovery is the rule and that the only people who have found persistent behavioral changes are the Cornell group. This statement should be examined very carefully to see whether persistent changes have been seen by other groups. In Chapters 10 and 13 below we will hear from Maria Simonson, of Johns Hopkins, and James Smart, of the University of Manchester. Both groups have published several papers demonstrating long-term behavioral effects.

Levine is impressed by the resiliency of the central nervous system. How do we know the central nervous system is resilient to the effects of early malnutrition when we do not know for certain what are the important parameters of the central nervous system?

The fact that the development of a particular physiological parameter is accelerated seems to surprise Levine. How does one interpret the fact that the pituitary gland response is quite elevated and that the animal, therefore, has an elevated response to stress? Is that good for the animal or is that bad for the animal? I do not really know, but at this moment it seems a bit naive to suggest that since the development of the pituitary-adrenal stress system is enhanced by malnutrition, development in the more global sense of behavioral and cognitive development is not depressed.

I find it a bit puzzling that Levine should so vigorously attack the concept that malnutrition experienced early in development may have profound consequences later in life when he and others pioneered the research on the long-term effects of early stress and thus helped substantiate such a concept.

The questions and controversies are now becoming very clear. I hope with an accumulation of data and rational argument we will eventually be able to resolve them.

PART III

MALNUTRITION AND SUBPRIMATE BEHAVIOR

Maria Simonson **10**

Effects of Maternal Malnourishment, Development, and Behavior in Successive Generations in the Rat and Cat

Alteration of the course and outcome of pregnancy through nutritional manipulation dates back to Biblical times, and legends have unfolded throughout history as to the influence of the mother's diet upon the offspring. Yet scientific acceptance of the adverse effects of maternal malnutrition on the physiological, biochemical, and emotional status of the fetus has come only in the last several decades. The classical study of Brozek and Vaes,[4] as well as the contributions of Barnes et al.,[2] Levitsky,[22] Fraňková,[13] Chow,[6] Coursin,[9] and others, have shown the long-reaching consequences of various types of maternal malnourishment on development and behavior. The many complex variables which must be considered in relation to behavior and growth, such as genetic endowment and environmental stresses, have been clearly demonstrated by Denenberg and Morton,[11] Levine,[20] Ader,[1] Levitsky et al.,[23] Caldwell and Churchill,[5] and others. Moreover, Zamenhof et al.,[39] Winick and Noble,[38] Levine and Mullins,[21] Platt and Stewart,[26] and Dickerson and Dobbing[12] have shed considerable enlightenment on the mechanisms of these behaviors. While Habicht et al.[14] and Blackwell et al.[3] among others have progressed to studies on the effects of maternal diet on human progeny, experimentation using various animal species will continue to serve as a basis for advanced explorations with possible extrapolation to humans.

Studies designed to test the effects on the offspring of restrictions in maternal diet during pregnancy and lactation have been carried out in our department of biochemistry at The Johns Hopkins University since as early as 1954. That a 50 percent overall restriction in dietary intake imposed on the mother rat during gestation and lactation results in permanent growth stunting and abnormal metabolism of offspring despite adequate diet after weaning was demonstrated in several experiments conducted in the laboratory.[7, 19] Subsequently, we extended our studies to investigate the effects of maternal malnourishment on the neuromotor development and behavior of the rat progeny. Our findings and the methodologies of the various dietary manipulations and testing procedures that we used in these latter studies have been reported in detail.[16, 30, 32, 33] In the present overview, a number of the significant findings growing out of our longitudinal studies on the rat will be presented and briefly discussed as background for a more detailed description (heretofore unpublished) of our replication of these studies—extended to three generations—in a different species, the cat.

In a series of experiments we recorded the long-term effects on the progeny of mothers whose diets had been restricted by 50 percent overall. To determine its relative importance to the fate of the offspring, the period of nutritional insult to the mother was variously imposed: during both gestation and lactation, during gestation alone, and during lactation alone. In sum, overall dietary restriction of the mother rat during gestation and lactation resulted in growth stunting and retardation to neuromotor development[32] as well as impaired learning capability[30] of the progeny. Restrictions during gestation alone produced a slight deficit in growth, lesser degree of delayed neuromotor development,[32] heightened emotional behavior,[33] and decreased capability in learning.[30] Behavioral deficiencies (both in learning and in emotionality) did not improve significantly with age in progeny suffering either of the above two periods of nutritional insult. When maternal dietary restriction was imposed only during lactation, the offspring were growth stunted and slightly emotional, but showed no impairment in learning.[16]

Among the important implications for behavior suggested by these findings is that although differences following maternal restriction during gestation alone were smaller in magnitude than those following restriction during both gestation and lactation, the fact that the pups were fostered to mothers that had been adequately fed throughout pregnancy permits the inference that maternal undernutrition had induced a direct effect upon the rat fetus. Thus, dietary restriction during pregnancy may cause a depletion of maternal reserves which is *not* immediately correctable by the restoration of adequate feeding at delivery. The above findings, taken together with the diminished effects observed on progeny of mothers restricted during lactation alone, suggest that the nutritional status of the mother during gestation has the most profound effect on the mental development of the offspring.

These findings thus support the work of other investigators who have pointed to the existence of a critical period during the early stages of life in which malnutrition can provoke permanent damage.[5, 39] In a study conducted in our own laboratory, we found that increasing the protein intake during the third trimester of pregnant rats maintained on a low-protein diet during the first two trimesters, tended to normalize the birth weight, growth, and behavior of the pups as compared with performance of pups born of dams maintained on low protein throughout pregnancy.[15] Additionally, in studies of human infants, Stoch and Smythe[36] and Monckeberg[25] have shown restricted intellectual development resulting from early malnourishment.

Our longitudinal studies on the rat also suggest a number of factors that must be taken into account in experiments designed to assess the impact of maternal malnourishment on the behavior of offspring. Among the most significant of these are non-nutritional influences which may contribute to behavioral decrements observed, and the relationship between body weight and behavior.

One non-nutritional factor that may influence the behavior of the offspring is the combination of effects of the mother's conduct during lactation. Restricted mothers are not generally good mothers. They are preoccupied by the search for food and are highly irritable. It would be surprising if the behavioral development of the progeny were not, to some extent, influenced by such atypical conduct of the mother during lactation. Moreover, if pups are nursed by their own mothers it is not possible to attribute subsequently observed abnormalities to damage sustained during fetal life. Therefore, in our later studies in the cat, all of our control and experimental animals were cross-fostered to adequately fed mothers, with no mother nursing her own kit. This feature of design avoided the hungry-mother effect, and allowed control of litter size, a factor which might also influence behavioral development, above and beyond any nutritionally mediated effect.

That the mother's age could also influence behavior was shown when we studied the effect of low-protein diets on pups, controlling for mother's age.[29] Here we found that pups of very young mothers (6-week-old rats) showed deleterious effects on both behavior and birth weight, even when the mother had been fed adequate protein. In examining the subsequent reproductive behavior of the mothers, however, no carryover effects were found.

Another significant finding in our investigations on the rat was that the neuromotor delays and behavioral abnormalities found in progeny of mothers restricted during gestation alone were not accompanied by corresponding deficits in weight during the period of observation. Thus, the widely applied index of body weight would have revealed no impairment in the experimental progeny, which were statistically indistinguishable by this criterion throughout the period of observation (even though they subsequently failed to match the growth of their controls). It is clear from these experiments that normal growth per se does not exclude the presence of damage from an earlier nutritional stress.

Additional light was shed on the relationship between behavior and weight in two experiments that we conducted on the role of protein in affecting the fate of the rat progeny. The first[27] was a study of progeny of dams fed a diet adequate in protein but low in calories; the second[28] studied progeny of dams whose diet was restricted in protein but was adequate in calories. While progeny born to mothers restricted in calories alone were of low birth weight, evinced a moderately increased neonatal mortality, and developed at a slower rate than the normally fed controls, their behavior was essentially normal. When mothers were fed a diet low in protein but adequate calorically, however, their offspring, while evincing normal birth weight, show marked behavioral aberations. Thus the above studies reinforce our earlier findings that normal birth weight does not preclude behavioral impairment, and support widely accepted evidence of the critical role that protein, as a crucial nutrient, plays in determining behavior in the offspring.

In light of the lack of investigation into generation effects in proportion to other studies, it became of interest to investigate whether the permanent and progressive changes that we found in the psychological functions of the male rat would persist in subsequent generations who had been given nutritional rehabilitation. Two studies on protein-restricted rat progeny include the early work of Whitley et al.[37] on maze learning in two generations, and the recently published study by Stewart et al.,[35] who reported on weight, growth, and behavior in 12 generations of marginal protein deficiency. In their attempts to rehabilitate low-protein-fed rats, Cowley and Griesel[10] concluded that more than one generation must be fed on a high plane of nutrition before all effects of the low-protein diet are overcome. More recent work by Levitsky et al.,[23] however, showed that the carryover differed in importance from that attributed by Cowley and Griesel. In our laboratories[17] rats born to mothers that were fed poor-quality protein during gestation and lactation and were raised on the same diet for more than one generation, exhibited severely retarded growth and delayed mental and neuromotor development. Continuation of feeding poor-quality protein brought about inferior survival, which showed itself markedly in both the second and third generations. Although there was marked reduction in growth, and in mental and neuromotor development, the severity did not increase, at least up to the second generation.

While investigators in other species (including the dog,[34] pig,[24] fowl,[8] and nonhuman primate[18]) have found the effects of progeny of maternal protein-calorie deprivation similar to those obtained in our studies of the rat, we chose to conduct our generation studies on the cat rather than the primate or rat for two reasons. First, the cat requires more protein and has a higher metabolism than any other laboratory animal. And second, the reproductive system of the cat is such that with fertilization occurring five days after copulation, implantation is not completed for 14 days (spontaneous ovulation takes place 24 hours after coitus). Thus, we were able to place the mother on either an adequate or restricted diet immediately following successful mating, an important factor considering that so much stress has been placed on instituting the protein restriction prior to conception.

To render the genetic factor more knowledgeable, all cats used in our experiments were of the Gantt strain used in closed colony breeding since 1956. Female cats that had had primary estrus but had not been bred were selected as mothers on the basis of similar age and weight to exclude any too-early pregnancy effects. Females were on the average 1.5 to 1.8 years old and weighed 6.8 to 7.2 pounds. The colony males (1 for every 5 females) averaged 1.9 to 2.2 years old and weighed approximately 10 to 11 pounds. When behavior indicated successful mating, the females were placed in separate cages in the breeding room, with specific environmental factors, such as lights, noise, and especially handling, carefully controlled. Upon confirmation of pregnancy, cats were assigned to control and experimental groups. Experimentals were given 45 g of Purina Chow ad libitum daily, or 50 percent of the food normally consumed by pregnant mothers as shown by previous food intake studies. Water was supplied ad libitum for both groups.

Within 24 hours of birth all male kittens (the females were held for further studies of reproductive behavior) were nursed ad libitum by foster mothers who had had no previous dietary restriction. Litters were maintained at 4 kits to each foster mother to insure adequate nursing and maternal care. No mother nursed her own kit. To insure constancy of behavior and to eliminate competition in nursing, the experimental and control kits were not mixed in nursing litters. Upon 7 weeks of age, kittens were weaned, fed ad libitum, transferred to another room, and housed in individual adjoining mesh open cages to offset any closed-cage isolation effect. These same procedures were followed for second and third generation experimentals and controls, all of whom received nutritionally adequate diets at all times.

Weight curves were maintained for several years. Figure 10.1 shows the growth curve of kits during early life. At birth, the experimental cats were slightly smaller but rapidly caught up to control weight levels at weaning. Later, we found a small difference in body weight, but this was not statistically significant until maturity. A similar delayed growth activity was also observed in rat progeny of mothers whose diets had also been restricted by 50 percent.

To measure physical and mental development, at 5 days of age kits were placed in a modified Franková box,[32] a specially scaled clear lucite box marked off in squares, for 6 minutes daily until day 40 of age. Since it was possible to observe the mother during labor and delivery, measurements were begun within several minutes after birth. Figure 10.2 shows delays evident in early measurements of physical, neuromotor, and behavioral indices of development. Other measurements recorded but not shown here in which experimental kits showed delay were: coloration density; pilo-erection; orienting and startle reflexes; and free fall righting response and mouse attack behavior. Experimental kits also lagged significantly behind the controls in manipulation of

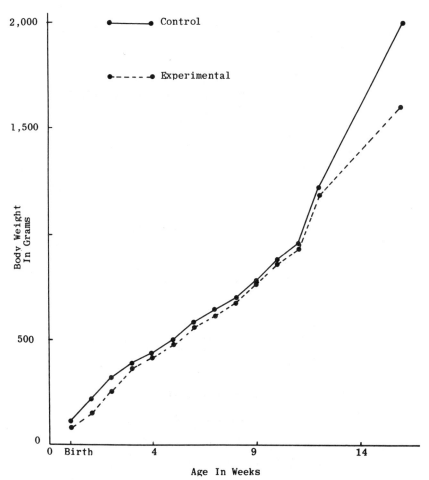

Figure 10.1. Growth of normal and gestation-restricted cats

objects and use of litter pans. Delays in exploratory activity were most striking, with experimentals lagging behind controls by a third. We found significant differences in all of these developmental indices similar to those reported in our rats. The greatest delays, both in magnitude and number, occurred at a later age, and seemed to correlate with the coordination necessary to

139

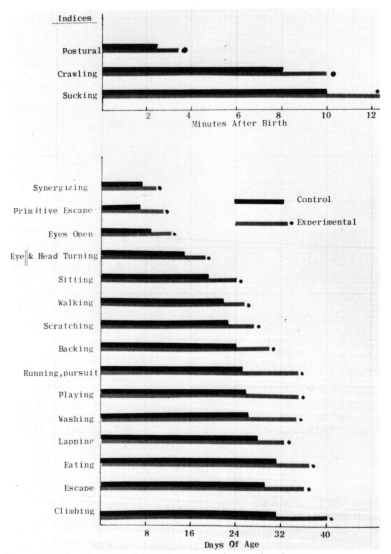

Figure 10.2. Development of normal and gestation-restricted cats

achieve the task. In our second generation, the delays were of far less magnitude and fewer in number, but obvious nevertheless. While dietary restriction had no significant effect on a number of responses, the type of response was often inappropriate. No neurological abnormalities were seen in the second generation, and our third-generation animals showed no significant differences in any of our developmental indices.

Replication of studies of social behavior conducted on our rats with like dietary backgrounds revealed similar results in the cat, including marked antisocial group interaction, abnormal posturings, and fluctuating dominant-submissive behavior in the prenatally malnourished cats that were clearly unlike the results observed in the controls. Dramatic effects seen in the first-generation experimental group are shown in Table 10.1. When in a group and a toy is introduced, control animals socialize and play. Experimental animals, however, are scared and/or aggressive—they vo-

Table 10.1. Summary

	First generation	Second generation	Third generation
Growth	Retarded at birth but approximated control weight within short period. Significant spread occurred about 4 to 5 months persisting throughout lifetime.	Slightly smaller at birth but rapidly achieved control weight with permanent maintenance	Equal to controls
Development	Delayed in all measurements	A very slight delay in some of the measurements	No delays
Learning	Decrements ranging from moderate to severe in all experiments	Same as control except for significant differences in maze reversal study	Equal to controls
Activity	Decreased	Normal	Normal
Emotionality	Heightened— significant	Moderate	Moderate
Neuromotor abnormalities	Significant in all experiments	None	None

calize, hiss, spit, and their pupils dilate; some show tremors, piloerection, and urination. Second-generation experimental cats were more antisocial in behavior than controls but did not display the excessive aggressive tendencies seen in generation one. In the third generation, there were no comparable differences.

Several problem-solving experiments were used to investigate another primary capacity, learning. A food-deprivation period of 24 hours was given to our 3.5-month-old kits, and measurements were obtained on various stages of learning: initial learning, relearning and after a 30-day period, extinction, and maze pattern reversal. Figure 10.3 shows the results of initial learning and reversal tasks. Again, controls were significantly superior to the experimental group in all measurements. The graph at the bottom of Figure 10.3 shows the errors made during the various stages of learning. Controls became totally error free in 11 trials, whereas our experimental cats had errors in all trials, but most markedly in the reversal pattern studies. Control animals quickly mastered new patterns of running the maze, but this was never achieved by the experimental group for whom such emotional behavior as urination, vocalization, and tremors also occurred with more frequency and intensity in this phase of the experiment. Indeed, the disruption of learned behavior by the simple substitution of new maze patterns and the marked difficulties of the experimental animals in achieving former performance levels leads to the speculation that they might be incapable of ever learning new tasks quite as well as control animals. Our second-generation animals obtained the same measurement levels in learning in all phases as controls until the reversal-pattern study where a complete disorganization and disruption of behavior occurred: the emotional behavior was significantly different, and the number of errors significantly higher. It took the experimentals considerably longer to run the maze, and they never achieved error-free trials. No dramatic neuromotor abnormalities appeared in this generation, however, and our third-generation cats showed no significant differences in any of their learning measurements or in their emotional behavior associated with learning.

To study emotional reaction and adaptation to environment, we measured reaction time and exploratory activity using open-field studies. The large wood arena with a detention arena (scaled to species) and floor marked in squares allowed complete visibility through a one-way glass window.[33] Twenty trials (ten minutes per

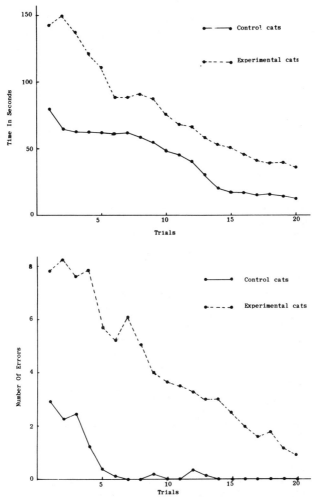

Figure 10.3. Top: Mean number of errors per trial of normal and gestation-restricted cats in learning initial maze problem. Bottom: Mean number of errors of same groups in learning maze reversal problem.

trial) were given each animal every other day. The results are shown in Figure 10.4. We found significant differences between experimentals and controls, indicating a possible delay in adaptation to environment. Many fear responses and other emotional behavior (as measured by the number of fecal boli) occurred in the experimental kits. There was a decrease in number of total squares entered as evidenced by door returns. Exploratory activity decreased as vocalization, urination, clawing, or circling increased, and they did not utilize the time allotted for activity. Differences were also observed in other tests administered, including conditioned emotional response (CER), visual cliff, discrimination, maze, avoidance behavior, social behavior, and other problem-solving tasks. In all of the above, no differences in either second- or third-generation cats were observed.

In summary, our experiments showed that a 50 percent overall dietary restriction of the mother during gestation results in significant damage to the growth, neuromotor development, and behavior of the offspring in both the rat and the cat, even though the birth weight of experimentals approximated that of controls at the time of measurement. Despite dietary rehabilitation, delays in development, learning decrements, and heightened emotionality, albeit less severe, persisted in our second-generation cats. By the third generation, experimentals were equal to controls in all indices except emotionality, in which they differed moderately but not significantly.

Our experiments represent the first study of maternal malnourishment in cats,[31] as well as the first generation studies of malnourished cats. While we did not attempt to investigate the mechanisms of these behaviors, some of our findings do suggest avenues for future investigations. Thus, Bacon Chow, finding that the pituitary glands of malnourished rats were smaller than those of controls, reasoned that this may have contributed to behavioral abnormalities in the rat. Shortly before his death Chow completed an experiment in which administration of pituitary extract corrected some of the animals' behaviors. Moreover, we found in our studies on rats, that the addition of protein to the maternal diet mimics somewhat the effect seen when progeny of dams subjected to 50 percent overall dietary restriction are treated with pituitary extracts.[28] One might argue that some of the added protein may be used to produce pituitary hormones or those hormones governing or governed by the pituitary. The above remains speculation, however, and more sophisticated experiments will be required to

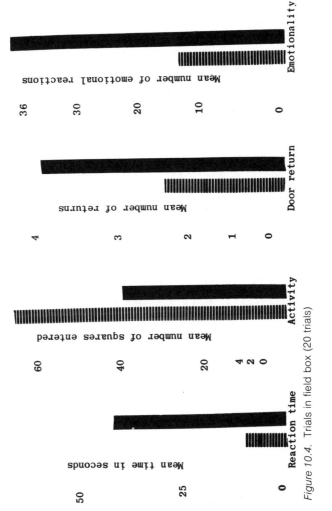

Figure 10.4. Trials in field box (20 trials)

direct our way to understanding such complex relationships as well as to determine their implications for human development and behavior.

References

1. Ader, R. The effects of early experience on subsequent emotionality and resistance to stress. *Psychol. Monogr.* 73 (No. 472): 1, 1959.
2. Barnes, R. H., S. R. Cunnold, R. R. Zimmermann, H. Simmons, R. B. MacLeod, and L. Krook. Influence of nutritional deprivations in early life on learning behavior of rats as measured by performance in a water maze. *J. Nutr.* 89: 399, 1966.
3. Blackwell, R. Q., B. F. Chow, K. S. K. Chinn, B. N. Blackwell, and S. C. Hsu. Prospective maternal nutrition study in Taiwan: Rationale, study design, feasibility, and preliminary findings. *Nutr. Reports Internat.* 7: 517, 1973.
4. Brozek, J., and G. Vaes. Experimental investigations on effects of dietary deficiency on animal and human behavior. *Vitam. Hormones* 19: 43, 1961.
5. Caldwell, D. F., and J. A. Churchill. Learning ability in the progeny of rats administered a protein-deficient diet during the second half of gestation. *Neurol.* 17: 95, 1967.
6. Chow, B. F. Effect of maternal nutrition on the development of the offspring. *Nutr. Reports Internat.* 7: 247, 1973.
7. Chow, B. F., and C. J. Lee, Effects of dietary restriction of pregnant rats on body weight gain of the offspring. *J. Nutr.* 82: 10, 1964.
8. Collier, G. H., and R. L. Squibb. Malnutrition and the learning capability of the chicken. In *Malnutrition, Learning, and Behavior*, N. S. Scrimshaw and J. E. Gordon, eds., M.I.T. Press, Cambridge, Mass., 1968, p. 236.
9. Coursin, D. B. Vitamin deficiencies and developing mental capacity. In *Malnutrition, Learning, and Behavior*, N. S. Scrimshaw and J. E. Gordon, eds., M.I.T. Press, Cambridge, Mass., 1968, p. 289.
10. Cowley, J. J., and R. D. Griesel. The development of second-generation low-protein rats. *J. Genet. Psychol.* 104: 89, 1964.
11. Denenberg, V. H., and J. R. C. Morton. Effects of environmental complexity and social groupings upon modification of emotional behavior. *J. Comp. Physiol. Psychol.* 55: 242, 1962.
12. Dickerson, J. W. T., and J. Dobbing. The effect of undernutrition early in life on the brain and spinal cord in pigs. *Proc. Nutr. Soc.* 26: 5, 1967.
13. Fraňková, S. Influence of a changed dietary pattern on the behavior of rats with a different excitability of the CNS. *Cs. Psychol.* 10: 13, 1966.
14. Habicht, J-P., C. Yarbrough, A. Lechtig, and R. E. Klein. Relationship of birth weight, maternal nutrition, and infant mortality. *Nutr. Reports Internat.* 7: 533, 1973.

15. Hsueh, A. M., M. Simonson, H. M. Hanson, and B. F. Chow. Protein supplementation to pregnant rats during third trimester and the growth arid behavior of offspring. *Nutr. Reports Internat.* 9: 31, 1974.
16. Hsueh, A. M., M. Simonson, M. J. Kellum, and B. F. Chow. Perinatal undernutrition and the metabolic and behavioral development of the offspring. *Nutr. Reports Internat.* 7: 437, 1973.
17. Hsueh, A. M., M. Simonson, M. J. Kellum, and B. F. Chow. Effect of poor quality protein on the growth and development of successive generation of rats. Unpublished study report. Department of Biochemistry, The Johns Hopkins School of Hygiene and Public Health, and Department of Psychiatry and Behavioral Sciences, The Johns Hopkins University School of Medicine, Baltimore, Maryland, 1973.
18. Kerr, G. R., and H. A. Waisman. A primate model for the quantitative study of malnutrition. In *Malnutrition, Learning, and Behavior*, N. S. Scrimshaw and J. E. Gordon, eds., M.I.T. Press, Cambridge, Mass., 1968, p. 240.
19. Lee, C. J., and B. F. Chow. Protein metabolism in the offspring of underfed mother rats. *J. Nutr.* 87: 439, 1965.
20. Levine, S. The effects of differential infantile stimulation on emotionality at weaning. *Canad. J. Psychol.* 13: 243, 1959.
21. Levine, S., and R. J. Mullins, Jr. Neonatal androgen or estrogen treatment and the adrenal cortical response to stress in adult rats. *Endocri.* 80: 1177, 1967.
22. Levitsky, D. Malnutrition and animal models of cognitive development. Proc. Kittay Scientific Foundation, in *Nutrition and Mental Functions*, George Serban, ed., Plenum Press, New York, 1975.
23. Levitsky, D., T. Massaro, and R. H. Barnes. Maternal malnutrition and the neonatal environment. *Fed. Proc.* 34(7): 1583, 1975.
24. Lowrey, R. S., W. G. Pond, R. H. Barnes, L. Krook, and J. K. Loosli. Influence of caloric level and protein quality on the manifestations of protein deficiency in the young pig. *J. Nutr.* 78: 245, 1962.
25. Monckeberg, F. Effect of early marasmic malnutrition on subsequent physical and psychological development. In *Malnutrition, Learning, and Behavior*, N. S. Scrimshaw and J. E. Gordon, eds., M.I.T. Press, Cambridge, Mass., 1968, p. 269.
26. Platt, B. S., and R. J. C. Stewart. The central nervous system of pigs on low-protein diets. *Proc. Nutr. Soc.* 19: viii, 1960.
27. Rider, A. A., and M. Simonson. Effect on rat offspring of maternal diet deficient in calories but not in protein. *Nutr. Reports Internat.* 7: 361, 1973.
28. Rider, A. A., and M. Simonson. The relationship between maternal diet, birth weight, and behavior of the offspring in the rat. *Nutr. Reports Internat.* 10: 19, 1974.
29. Rider, A. A., and M. Simonson. Characteristics of very young mother rats and their pups on low protein diets. *Nutr. Reports Internat.* 10: 345, 1974.

30. Simonson, M., and B. F. Chow. Maze studies on progeny of underfed mother rats. *J. Nutr.* 100: 685, 1970.

31. Simonson, M., H. M. Hanson, L. M. Roeder, and B. F. Chow. Effects of growth hormones and pituitary extract on behavioral abnormalities in offspring of undernourished rats. *Nutr. Reports Internat.* 7: 321, 1973.

32. Simonson, M., R. W. Sherwin, J. K. Anilane, W. Y. Yu, and B. F. Chow. Neuromotor development in progeny of underfed mother rats. *J. Nutr.* 98: 18, 1969.

33. Simonson, M., J. K. Stephen, H. M. Hanson, and B. F. Chow. Open field studies in offspring of underfed mother rats. *J. Nutr.* 101: 331, 1971.

34. Stewart, R. J. C., and B. S. Platt. Nervous system damage in experimental protein-calorie deficiency. In *Malnutrition, Learning, and Behavior*, N. S. Scrimshaw and J. E. Gordon, eds., M.I.T. Press, Cambridge, Mass., 1968, p. 168.

35. Stewart, R. J. C., R. F. Preece, and H. G. Sheppard. Twelve generations of marginal protein deficiency. *Brit. J. Nutr.* 33: 233, 1975.

36. Stoch, M. B., and P. M. Smythe. Undernutrition during infancy, and subsequent brain growth and intellectual development. In *Malnutrition, Learning, and Behavior*, N. S. Scrimshaw and J. E. Gordon, eds., M.I.T. Press, Cambridge, Mass., 1968, p. 278.

37. Whitley, J. R. B., B. L. O'Dell, and A. G. Hogan. Effect of diet on maze learning in second-generation rats: Folic acid deficiency. *J. Nutr.* 45: 153, 1951.

38. Winick, M., and A. Noble. Cellular response in rats during malnutrition at various ages. *J. Nutr.* 89: 300, 1966.

39. Zamenhof, S., E. Van Marthens, and L. Grauel. DNA (cell number) and protein in neonatal rat brain: Alteration by timing of maternal dietary protein restriction. *J. Nutr.* 101: 1265, 1971.

Slávka Fraňková **11**

Behavioral Consequences of Early Malnutrition and Environmental Stimuli

The performance of behavioral experiments on malnourished animals has become almost fashionable and a relatively easy way to collect material for a Ph.D. thesis. The beginner approaches the study of interactions between behavior and malnutrition with great optimism and enthusiasm, eager to measure activity in the open field, defecation at the same place, rate of learning in the maze or in the shuttle box, and further behavioral features, the battery of tests being dependent on the availability of equipment in the laboratory. He is satisfied with his work because it is very easy to reveal significant differences between control and nutritionally deprived groups. The first skepticism and doubts come when comparing one's own findings with those of equally serious authors who report contradictory results. The number of controversies gradually increases and this results in pessimism and distrust for work that brings so many problems and uncertainties. In our research we have been trying to find answers to such questions as: Does early malnutrition result in the deterioration of processes of memory, learning, and intelligence? Does spontaneous activity of the malnourished or rehabilitated animal increase or decrease? Is it possible to make any extrapolation from animal to man?

Our experimental work at the Institute of Human Nutrition, Prague, Czechoslovakia, on behavioral responses to different nutritional plans started in 1958. Influenced by the findings of Lát,[16,17] we compared behavioral effects of increased dietary levels of fats, carbohydrates, or proteins in adult animals. Changes in spontaneous exploratory activity and in avoidance learning were evident in the course of the dietary treatment.[5,6] Logically, the next step led to the effect of dietary changes occurring earlier in life.

We decided to observe the development of spontaneous behavior under different nutritional plans during the first weeks of life. The description of behavioral development by Bolles and Woods[2] helped us design our method. Beginning on day 3 of life we tested the first appearance and frequency of different activities performed in a new environment by pups reared in small litters (4 pups per litter), or in larger litters (13 pups per litter). We expected a higher activity level in small litters that would be in agreement with the findings of Lát, Widdowson, and McCance,[18] who reported accelerated neural and behavioral development in fast-growing overnourished pups. However, we failed to demonstrate the difference between over- and undernourished groups (Figure 11.1).

We were not sure what was wrong and therefore repeated the experiment with a larger number of experimental groups and litters with 4, 9, 13, or 17 pups. We observed somewhat more rapid development in litters of 9 and 13, but slower in both small and extremely large litters.[8] These results were disappointing again—the rats consistently refused to behave as we had expected.

Levine's articles on psychophysiological effects of early handling came at just the right time.[20,21] Previously, psychological research and nutritional research on postnatal development had been done separately. From Levine's results, it appeared that early nutrition must be considered but one link in the chain of interactions between the developing organism and stimuli from the external environment. While in most experimental designs, environment had been considered a constant factor and had therefore been neglected, it was now apparent that, on the contrary, external environment must be included in the experimental design as one of the most important variables.

Since it was highly probable that the behavioral effect of litter size was masked in our experiments by the everyday manipulation with pups, we tested the hypothesis that external stimulation was the factor modifying the effects of early malnutrition.

On testing the intensity of exploratory activity in rats not handled until day 90 of life, we found an inverse relationship between litter size and frequency of rearing (Figure 11.2). Regular handling modified the effect of early nutrition, as manipulated by litter size,

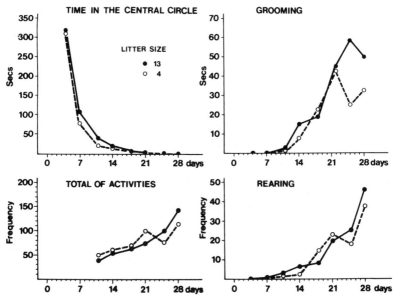

Figure 11.1. Behavioral development in pups reared in large or small litters. Pups were placed in the middle of the observing box. Characteristics were recorded: time to leave the central area (a circle, 10 cm in diameter, drawn on the floor), time spent with grooming, frequency of various spontaneous activities, and rearing performed during 6 minutes of observation.

and resulted in increased exploratory activity in all groups. The handled undernourished pups did not differ from control rats, reared in litters of medium size, that were not handled.

We found a beneficial effect of early handling also in prematurely weaned males and in rats whose mothers were food-restricted during lactation.[8] The results were reported in 1966 at the International Congress of Nutrition in Hamburg,[7] and at the Conference on Malnutrition, Learning, and Behavior at M.I.T. in 1967.[8] But a serious question remained: Why did the quantitative effect of constant stimulation vary in litters of different size? When the experimental design was analyzed it appeared that actually more than two variables (nutrition and a defined amount of stimulation by the experimenter) played a part. The effect of each external stimulation on an individual was mediated through the changes in the whole system—the family. Different litter size meant, logically, different psychological conditions both for pups

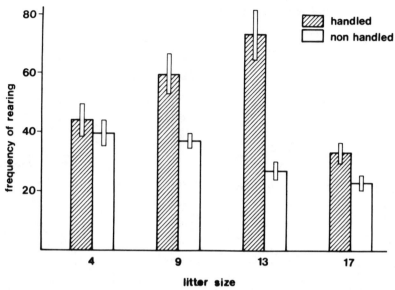

Figure 11.2. Exploratory activity in adult male rats, reared in litters of 4, 9, 13, or 17 pups. Frequency of rearing was tested in groups of rats, either handled during the preweaning period or left undisturbed until day 90 of life. Exploratory activity was tested in the open field during 10 minutes on days 91, 100, and 110. Values of these 3 tests were combined.

and their mother. Thus, in the small family, mutual stimulation was low, and intervention did not substantially influence behavior of the members of the family. In a litter with 17 pups, however, the number of mutual contacts was originally high, and further manipulation with the nest could result in the overstimulation of pups and disturb the mother as well.

It became evident that we needed more information about the interactions between early nutrition and the psychological and social situations within the family, about the responses of the mother to nutritional deprivation and feedback from pups, and about the effect on various environmental stimuli.

During the following years we studied the effect of malnutrition on the lactating dam, behavioral development of pups, later behavioral effects, interactions within the family, and increased or decreased sensorial stimulation. In most of the experiments we used the model of protein-calorie deprivation, introduced by Barnes.[1]

First, we turned our attention to the lactating dam, supposing she had the key position in the chain of interactions. At the beginning, the mother is the exclusive donator of nutrients and the source of sensorial stimuli. Rosenblatt demonstrated the synchronization between maternal behavior and the behavior of the developing pup.[27]

We tested the behavior of lactating females in various experimental set-ups. In the first experiment we found decreased retrieving activity, lower score for maternal activities, and more exploration during the test interval in those females fed on a low-protein diet (Figure 11.3).[10] These results were confirmed by observations of Smart and Preece.[29] Recently,[12] we observed maternal behavior in more detail, being especially interested in the adaptation of mothers to changed external environment. The mother with pups was inserted into a complex maze, and, during the standard time interval, arrangement of a new nest, latency to the first contact, frequency and duration of contacts with pups, and other activities performed in the maze were recorded. In all criteria, the protein-deprived dams were inferior to the normally fed rats (Figure 11.4). We preferred this type of observation to the simple recording of events in the breeding cage. It seemed to correspond better to natural living conditions, where the lactating dam had often to leave the nest, seek food, transfer the pup to a safe place when necessary, and so on.

Massaro and Levitsky found that more time was spent in the nesting area by the protein-deprived mothers than by the controls.[24] Nevertheless, they also observed that the malnourished mothers performed more rearing activity in this situation. These observations were similar to those described in our paper[10] and in that of Smart and Preece.[29]

During the last 10 years we have tested behavioral development and later behavioral patterns in the early protein-deprived rats. We observed delayed development of spontaneous exploratory activities, disturbance in social behavior, and qualitatively different responses to various environmental conditions.[9,11,14,15] We felt, however, that the problem of early external stimulation remained open. The increased stimulation caused by handling potentiated the activity of calorically deprived rats. We were not successful, however, in using the handling technique in the protein-deprived pups. Each manipulation with the pups disturbed their mother so that she refused to return to her infants for a long time. Leathwood reported a negative effect in the handling

153

Slávka Fraňková

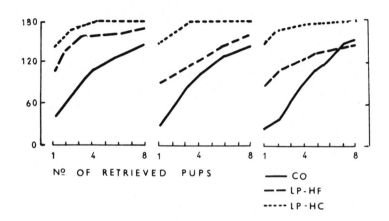

RATE OF RETRIEVING

Nº OF RETRIEVED PUPS

—— CO
— — LP-HF
····· LP-HC

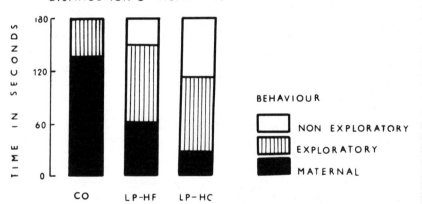

DISTRIBUTION OF ACTIVITIES

TIME IN SECONDS

CO   LP-HF   LP-HC

BEHAVIOUR

NON EXPLORATORY
EXPLORATORY
MATERNAL

Figure 11.3. Maternal behavior in the retrieving test. Time to retrieve eight pups and distribution of activities performed during 3 minutes of observation was recorded in groups fed on the control diet (solid line), low protein-high fat diet (barred line), and low protein-high carbohydrate diet (dotted line).

154

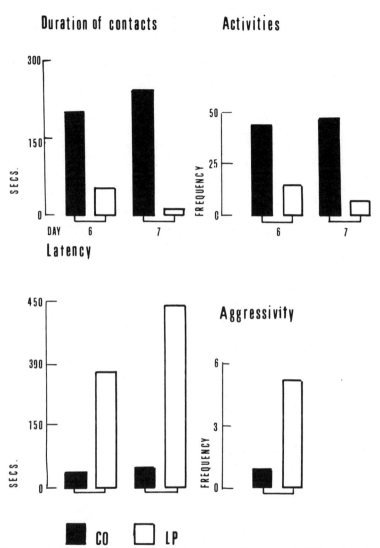

Figure 11.4. Behavior of lactated dams in a new environment. Activities of the lactated dams were measured during the 10 minutes of observation on day 6 and day 7 after the delivery. Black columns = control group; white columns = protein-deprived group.

of undernourished mice.[19] His handling, however, took place for 12 to 15 minutes daily, and it was probably accompanied with stress of separation from the mother and with possible cooling. The handled mice did not differ from the undernourished group in learning performance. Levitsky and Barnes[23] reported beneficial effects of handling in protein-deprived rats. In their experiment, however, the preweaning stimulation was followed by the postweaning one. The stimulated rats were housed in pairs, while the controls were kept in isolation. Under these conditions, it would not seem possible to make definite conclusions about behavioral effects of early stimulation.

To avoid technical problems of handling caused by a possible adverse effect of the experimenter and a negative effect on the lactating dam, we decided to stimulate the animals with one of their own kind. We were fascinated by the work of Denenberg et al.,[4] Plaut and Davis,[26] and Nováková and Šterc,[25] who reported beneficial effects of a rat "aunt" on the development and later behavior of rats or mice.

In one experiment, the lactating dams and their pups were assigned to two groups: control and protein-deprived. To one-half of each group of families the "aunts" were added to increase the social stimulation within the family. The aunts were adult virgin normal females trained to pups of different age ("sensitized" according to Rosenblatt[28]). The aunt spent the daytime with the family in the breeding cage and in the late afternoon was returned to her home cage and provided with food. The aunt continued visiting the family after weaning, until day 49 of life. Behavioral characteristics were observed in pups during the preweaning period, that is, spontaneous behavior and interactions with litter mates and with the mother. Contacts with alien pups and with their own pups were observed in female rats. The behavioral patterns of the malnourished pups did not differ from those of the control rats reared without the aunt.[13]

Levitsky[22] proposed the term "functional isolation" to characterize the psychology of the malnourished rat. There are several factors that might contribute to functional isolation of the protein-deprived animal. Behavioral abnormalities of the lactating mother could be the first factor responsible for behavioral disturbances of the infant. The mother does not stimulate the pups to activity, or, perhaps, does not respond properly to stimuli from the pup. The imprinting image and early experience with the mother are especially important for later maternal activities in the early malnourished females.

Second, the delayed motor and sensorial development during the critical developmental periods make it difficult to gain from experiences offered by the environment. The lack of energy results in decreased mutual contacts and feedback from litter mates. This results in further impoverishment of the environment. A kind of psychic deprivation could develop even in the large family, if affected by malnutrition.

The activity of the individual in seeking new stimuli is also an important factor. A normal infant looks for external stimuli in play, satisfied with any play material. The sick individual pays no attention to the most perfect and stimulating toys. Therefore, when designing the stimulation program for the deprived infant, it is necessary to take into account whether he is able to take advantage of the provided stimulation. The block could be morphological (unsatisfactory development of motor or sensorial apparatuses), or energetic (lack of available energy for physical activity and for mental effort), or central (qualitative ways of decoding or processing information). The last aspect is very puzzling and deserves more thought.

After consideration of the value of individual findings, controversies, and limiting and codetermining factors, persistent questions remain: What sort of animals are early-malnourished rats and in what behavioral patterns do they really differ?

Most of the experiments have been designed to answer simple questions, such as: How many stimuli does the malnourished rat need to solve the task designed? Is the spontaneous activity level higher or lower in the open field? Is the defecation score higher or lower in the type of observing box used? We were perfectly all right at the first stage of the study of behavior-nutrition interactions when asking these simple quantitative questions. All of us asked and solved the problems this way. But now, I believe, it is time to ask different questions. In 1973, DeLicardie and Cravioto presented an excellent paper at the World Health Organization Conference in Saltsjöbaden, Sweden.[3] They talked about their study of the behavioral style of malnourished children. They asked not *how well* but *how* they performed. This approach leads us to one of the roots of the problem. There is ample evidence and also general agreement that the malnourished individual (human

157

as well as animal) differs *qualitatively* from the normal one. He adapts in a different way to new environment, and he displays social interactions other than the normal and different spontaneous behavior under constant or changed environment. Qualitative changes and generally different responses to reality are the most striking features of the malnourished infant. We would design better experiments by thinking more in terms of basic common processes than by seeking too detailed results of an individual laboratory experiment.

We do not need to be pessimistic about the controversies between findings of different laboratory experiments. Similar situations exist in human research, too. A typical example is that of psychic deprivation during early childhood, which for some individuals may result in later schizophrenia, criminality, or neuroses while others remain clinically normal; so, too, some individuals will be well adapted to the social environment, others will be successful but not happy, and so on. This does not mean total skepticism toward the study of behavioral ontogeny or rejection of the hypothesis of the interaction between early deprivation and later behavioral disturbances.

It is most important for researchers working on an animal model to have the opportunity to discuss more often their problems with colleagues working in the related field of human development. It could be a reminder that even the laboratory experiment has to serve a most urgent problem: how to help children damaged by the injustice of a contemporary society that is incapable of satisfying the basal needs of the growing child.

References

1. Barnes, R. H., C. S. Neely, E. Kwong, B. A. Labadan, and S. Fraňková. Postnatal nutritional deprivation as determinants of adult behavior toward food, its consumption and utilization. *J. Nutr.* 96: 467, 1968.
2. Bolles, R. C., and P. J. Woods. The ontogeny of behaviour in the albino rat. *Anim. Behav.* 12: 427, 1964.
3. DeLicardie, E. R., and J. Cravioto. Behavioral responsiveness of survivors of clinical severe malnutrition to cognitive demands. In *Symp. Swedish Nutr. Found.*, XII, Almqvist and Wiksell, Uppsala, 1974, p. 134.
4. Denenberg, V., G. A. Hudgens, and M. X. Zarrow. Mice reared with rats: Effects of mother on adult behavior patterns. *Psychol. Rep.* 18: 451, 1966.
5. Fraňková, S. Relationship between dietary fat intake and higher nervous activity in rats. *Activ. Nerv. Super.*, Prague, 4: 471, 1962.

6. Fraňková, S. Influence of a changed dietary pattern on the behaviour of rats with a different excitability of the CNS. *Cs. Psychol.* 10: 13, 1966.

7. Fraňková, S. Influence of nutrition and stimulation in early infancy on exploratory behavior of adult rats. *Proc. 7th Internat. Congr. Nutr.*, Hamburg, 1966, Pergamon Press 5: 11, 1967.

8. Fraňková, S. Nutritional and psychological factors in the development of spontaneous behavior in the rat. In *Malnutrition, Learning, and Behavior*, N. S. Scrimshaw and J. E. Gordon, eds., M.I.T. Press, Cambridge, Mass., 1968, p. 312.

9. Fraňková, S. Late sequences of early nutritional and sensoric deprivations in rats. *Activ. Nerv. Super.* 12: 155, 1970.

10. Fraňková S. Relationship between nutrition during lactation and maternal behaviour of rats. *Activ. Nerv. Super.* 13: 1, 1971.

11. Fraňková, S. Effect of protein calorie malnutrition on the development of social behavior in rat. *Devel. Psychobiol.* 6: 33, 1973.

12. Fraňková, S. Effects of protein deficiency in early life and during lactation on maternal behaviour. *Baroda J. Nutr.* (India) 1: 21, 1974.

13. Fraňková, S. Influence of early social environment on behavior of the protein-calorie malnourished rats. *Activ. Nerv. Super.* 16: 98, 1974.

14. Fraňková, S., and R. H. Barnes. Influence of malnutrition in early life on exploratory behavior of rats. *J. Nutr.* 96: 477, 1968.

15. Fraňková, S., and R. H. Barnes. Effect of malnutrition in early life on avoidance conditioning and behavior of adult rats. *J. Nutr.* 96: 485, 1968.

16. Lát, J. On mythical average organism and on the significance of interindividual (constitutional, biological) variability. *Cs. fysiol.* 7: 97, 1958 (in Czech).

17. Lát, J., and E. Faltová. Effects of various level of animal proteins on higher nervous activity of rats. *Cs. fysiol.* 4: 171, 1955 (in Czech).

18. Lát, J., E. M. Widdowson, and R. A. McCance. Some effects of accelerating growth. III. Behaviour and nervous activity. *Proc. Roy. Soc. Biol.* 153: 347, 1961.

19. Leathwood, P. D., M. S. Bush, and J. Mauron. The effects of chlordiazepoxide on avoidance performance of mice subjected to undernutrition or handling stress in early life. *Psychopharm.* 41: 105, 1975.

20. Levine, S. Psychophysiological effects of infantile stimulation. In *Roots of Behavior*, E. L. Bliss, ed., Hoeber, New York, 1962, p. 246.

21. Levine, S., and M. Alpert. Differential maturation of the central nervous system as a function of early experience. *Arch. Gen. Psychiat.* 1: 403, 1959.

22. Levitsky, D. A. Malnutrition and animal models of cognitive development. Proc. Kittay Scientific Foundation, in *Nutrition and Mental Functions*, George Serban, ed., Plenum Press, New York, 1975, p. 75.

23. Levitsky, D. A., and R. H. Barnes. Nutritional and environmental interactions in the behavioral development of the rat: Long-term effects. *Science* 176: 68, 1972.

Slávka Fraňková

24. Massaro, T. F., D. A. Levitsky, and R. H. Barnes. Protein malnutrition in the rat: Its effects on maternal behavior and pup development. *Devel. Psychobiol.* 7: 551, 1974.
25. Nováková, V., and J. Šterc. Late effects of early hunger and mother-litter separation on learning and memory in male rats. *Physiol. Behav.* 11: 277, 1973.
26. Plaut, S. M., and J. M. Davis. Effects of mother-litter separation on survival, growth and brain amino acid levels. *Physiol. Behav.* 8: 43, 1972.
27. Rosenblatt, J. S. The basis of synchrony in the behavioral interaction between the mother and her offspring in the laboratory rat. In *Determinants of Infant Behaviour*, III, B. M. Foss, ed., Methuen, London, 1965.
28. Rosenblatt, J. S. Nonhormonal basis of maternal behavior in the rat. *Science* 156: 1512, 1973.
29. Smart, J. L., and J. Preece. Maternal behaviour of undernourished mother rat. *Anim. Behav.* 21: 613, 1973.

David A. Levitsky **12**

Malnutrition and the Hunger to Learn

In 1956, Geber and Dean published a paper in which they reported significant retardation in intellectual and developmental measures in children who had suffered severe protein and calorie malnutrition.[10] This was an important finding not only because it pointed out another handicap for the young developing nations, but because it brought the problem of behavior and cognitive development to the attention of nutritional scientists who had long been primarily concerned with problems of physiology and biochemistry.

One of the first of the nutritional scientists who foresaw the significance of this problem and had the courage to pursue research in this area was Richard H. Barnes, who, wise in the ways of research, knew that nutritionists alone could not make a significant contribution to this area, and so engaged psychologists to work with him in his research on malnutrition and behavioral development. His first major paper on this subject was published in the *Journal of Nutrition* in 1966. Among its authors were two nutritionists, three psychologists, and one physiologist. In that now-famous paper there were several very important observations: first, malnutrition inflicted in early life, but followed by nutritional rehabilitation, produced a long-term effect on adult behavior; second, the effect was considerably greater in males than in females; and finally, one of the most obvious behavioral differences was in "emotionality." The authors suggested that perhaps the apparent "learning" differences observed may have been due to this difference in emotionality.

Barnes was joined by Slávka Fraňková, from the Institute of Human Nutrition, Prague. Fraňková had been a student of Josef Lát, a well-recognized psychologist in Europe who had developed very sensitive techniques for detecting behavioral changes. Along with Lát, Fraňková had demonstrated that these techniques could

161

reliably detect behavioral differences induced by diet. Combining the sophistication in behavioral measurement of Fraňková with the well-designed nutritional methodology of Barnes, papers were published in the *Journal of Nutrition* which again confirmed the long-term behavioral effects of early malnutrition.[3,9]

These papers raised some other important questions. First, they showed that the feeding behavior of the adult rat was affected by early malnutrition.[3] This was of particular significance to those using food as reinforcement when studying the effects of early malnutrition on learning. Second, they observed open-field behavior to be quite sensitive to the effects of early malnutrition. Third, in tests of avoidance conditioning, no effect of early malnutrition on the rate of avoidance conditioning was observed, although rats malnourished early in life extinguished significantly more slowly. Finally, they pointed out that the previously malnourished rats appeared more "emotional"—requiring more trials to extinguish to the conditioned stimulus and displaying more intertrial behavior than controls.

I joined Barnes in 1968, soon after Fraňková returned to Czechoslovakia. From the onset, I shared Barnes's enthusiasm over the possibility of creating a model of behavioral and cognitive retardation in animals. We were strongly influenced by the work of Myron Winick in New York and John Dobbing in England who demonstrated the susceptibility of certain periods of early development to severe nutritional insult of the organism. Specifically, they observed that a period of malnutrition at the time of rapid brain growth produced long-term irreversible depression in "brain cells" as measured by DNA content. Although behavioral studies were few at this time as documented in the proceedings of the 1967 M.I.T. Conference,[26] the concept emerged that it was this depression in brain cells which caused mental retardation. The concept is a mechanistic one, that is, it is the irreversible damage to the neural hardware that is causing the problem.

Although I was stimulated by the possibility of creating a model of mental retardation through nutritional insult, I was also aware of the work of Karl Lashley, published in the early 1930's, in which he demonstrated that following fairly extensive destruction to brain tissue very early in the life of young mammals, it was difficult to demonstrate alterations in problem-solving ability in the adult.[15]

It is important, at this point, to review the status of animal models of cognitive development held at that time. The major method of assessing cognitive function in the animal was, and still is today, the measurement of the rate of problem solving. The conventional technique is to deprive the animal of a nutrient, place the animal in a situation in which a distinct set of stimuli are presented, and observe the rate of responding correctly to presented stimuli. If the organism responds correctly to the stimuli that the experimenter deems important, it receives the wanted nutrient. There are several variations of this method. One may use an aversive stimuli instead of nutrient deficiency to induce a solution. Instead of observing the rate of solving a particular problem, one may observe the rate of learning of a series of problems (learning sets) or the rate of unlearning one solution and learning another (reversal or nonreversal shifts). However, all these methods have one feature in common: the experimenter always *directs* the animal as to what to learn, by making the reinforcement always contingent upon attending to the appropriate stimuli. Almost all of the animal work in the fields of both developmental and comparative psychology utilized this "directed" learning paradigm for the assessment of cognitive processing.

One of the major problems in assessing learning is that we cannot measure learning directly. We are permitted only to observe the effects of learning as expressed in the performance of an organism. Moreover, there are many factors that may affect the performance of an organism in a learning situation which may not affect the learning process at all. Thus, in order to make a valid conclusion that a decrease in learning performance of an animal reflects an impairment in the ability to learn, one must be able to rule out the possibility that the effects are due to performance factors.

There had been several reports in the literature purporting to show that malnutrition produced deficits in learning ability. After critically reviewing the literature, however, we concluded that most of these studies had failed to control adequately for possible performance factors.[20] Since we were interested ultimately in assessing the effect of malnutrition on cognitive processing, it was important that we understand as much as possible about the effects of early malnutrition on all those performance factors that might confound studies of learning in animals. Of these possible confounding performance factors, we were mostly concerned about food and water motivation and "emotional reactivity."

Table 12.1 is a summary of the results of several studies on

David A. Levitsky

Table 12.1. Food and water consumption

	Control	Experimental	P value
Rats			
Food consumed, gms/day/100 gm body weight	4.2	5.2	P < .001
Food consumed, gms/day/100 gm (body-weight)3/4	.205	.224	P < .01
Percent food spilled in 1-hour test	3.5	24.6	P < .001
Water consumed, ml/day/100 gm body weight	6.25	8.60	P < .001
Water (in food)	1.45	1.67	P < .01
Pigs			
Food consumed, gms/kg body weight/day	29.3	52.7	P < .01

feeding and drinking behavior in adult rats and pigs subject to severe malnutrition during postnatal development. Early malnutrition produced an increase in the food intake of rats and pigs and an increase in the water intake of rats, when intake is expressed as a ratio to body size. More critical to the argument of motivational influence, we found that when nutritionally rehabilitated rats were placed on a one-hour feeding schedule, they appeared hyperexcited and spilled a large percentage of their food, replicating an earlier observation by Barnes.[3]

This reaction is probably very closely related to early-deprivation induced-hoarding behavior, a phenomenon observed by Marx in the early 1950's.[22] Not only did the early-malnourished rat display a greater excitement when later deprived of food, but it also showed a greater motivation to eat as measured by rate of bar-pressing for food as a function of the percentage weight lost (see Figure 12.1). Thus, food and possibly water motivation of adult animals appeared altered by early malnutrition. Many of those studying the effects of early malnutrition recognized this possibility of altered appetitive motivation and tried to avoid the problem by using aversive conditioning procedures.

We then turned our attention to assessing the animal's reaction to aversive stimuli. Fraňková and Barnes[9] and Smart[28] demonstrated an effect on the open-field behavior of rats malnourished early in life. We substantiated this observation.[18,19] Table 12.2

164

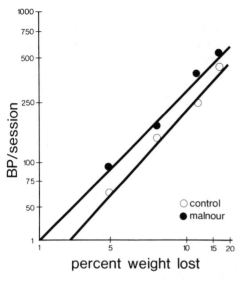

Figure 12.1. Mean total bar presses per session as a function of percent body weight loss for previously malnourished rats and controls

shows an increase in locomotor activity in rats and pigs malnourished early in life, then rehabilitated. The effect was most pronounced during the first 10 minutes of testing. After adaption to the apparatus, a difference in behavior of the postnatally malnourished animals and controls could be re-established if the animals were then startled by a loud sound. When startled in the open field the rats usually rushed into a corner, defecated, urinated, and squealed. All animals, regardless of early dietary con-

Table 12.2. Results of behavioral tests

	Control	Experimental	P value
Rats			
Open field (spontaneous activity)	51.9	76.9	P < .01
Response to loud sound (percent locomotor reduction)	56.0	74.3	P < .01
Passive avoidance (reciprocal latency)	.095	.020	P < .01
Sidman Avoidance Test (bar press per min.)	3.97	5.59	P < .01
Foot shock, flinch threshold (ma.)	.167	.143	P < .005
Pigs			
Open field (spontaneous activity)	33	72	P < .001

165

dition, appeared to behave similarly, although the previously malnourished animals maintained this immobile behavior for a longer duration than the well-nourished controls, suggesting an exaggerated response to the aversive stimulus, the loud noise.

Another example of this increased responsiveness to aversive stimuli can be seen in rats placed in a step-down test of passive avoidance. If an animal previously malnourished was placed on a small platfoform, its initial latency to leave the platform was no different than the behavior of controls. If, after stepping off the platform, the animal was given a brief electric shock and replaced on the platform, then the latency to leave the platform the second time was significantly greater than that of controls. It is unfortunate that we did not run a nonshocked control group in this study to assess whether the effect was due to a reaction to the electric shock, as we interpreted, or due to retesting. I believe we were lucky in correctly interpreting the response as an increased reaction to the aversive stimulus, since subsequent experiments have confirmed the effect in other situations. For example, we have observed that previously malnourished rats respond at a greater rate to avoid an electric shock as measured in a Sidman Avoidance Test. Moreover, in more recent experiments, we found the threshold for a behavior response of the early malnourished rat to an electric shock to be significantly lower than that of controls (Table 12.2). Thus, we concluded that both motivational and emotional factors are affected by early malnutrition—a matter which makes the interpretation of learning experiments very difficult.

How then could one measure rate of learning in the previously malnourished animal? One solution was found by George Collier,[4] who devised a test situation in which the animal presents itself with a problem. The rate of problem presentation can be used as an index motivation, and the probability of a correct choice is the index of learning. We modified this technique by selecting a rate of bar pressing (motivation) to which we made all animals perform before testing learning. We accomplished this by adjusting the amount of food we fed each animal following testing.[17] Thus, if the animal's rate of responding was below our criterion, we gave the animal less food following testing. On the subsequent test, the bar-pressing rate was usually higher. After reaching stable rates the animals were presented with a two-choice, noncorrection, visual-discrimination problem.

166

Figure 12.2 shows the number of correct choices per 50 trials for a group of rats malnourished early in life and their controls. There is no evidence of any difference in rate of learning. No difference in the rate of learning was observed in the reversal problem. We then instituted an alternative problem which required the animal to alternate between two bars in order to obtain a reinforcement. A slight difference in performance was noted. We then instituted a minimum of 15 seconds between trials in the situation. Figure 12.3 shows the results. There was a significant difference in alternation behavior; the previously malnourished animals displayed poorer performance than controls. We originally thought we had discovered a deficit in short-term memory, but close inspection of the response record showed the previously malnourished animals took a significantly longer latency to present the problem following an error than controls. We interpreted this last test as possibly illustrating an emotional reaction to the no-reward situation. The results of the alternation tests are important only in that they showed our experimental procedures were sensitive enough to detect a behavioral difference due to early malnutrition, yet no differences could be observed in the rate of learning the visual-discrimination problem in our controlled-motivation testing situation. We have repeated this study twice and have never observed any significant effect of early malnutrition on rate of learning

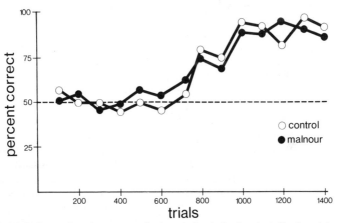

Figure 12.2 Group learning curve of original discrimination test. Each point represents mean percent correct responses averaged for 100 trials.

David A. Levitsky

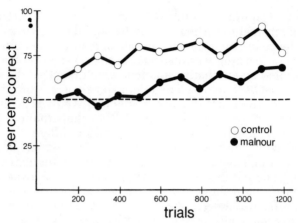

Figure 12.3. Group learning curve of 15 second delayed-alternation test

under conditions of controlled motivation. Thus, we concluded that early malnutrition does not impair the ability of an animal to learn visual stimulus-response associations.

At about this time we became increasingly aware of the possible relevance of another area of research. Denenberg[5] and Levine[16], for example, have demonstrated the powerful effect of early environment on later behavior in animals. Early stimulation produced by "handling" animals during lactation produced a long-term decrease in emotional "reactivity" when measured in the adult. R. Melzack and others found environmental "isolation" experienced very early in life increased the emotional reactivity of dogs.[24] What was most interesting to us was the observation that emotional reactivity was the primary behavioral domain which was affected by very early environmental stimulation. This is what we had observed in rats and pigs.

Melzack's explanation was based on the postulation that emotional reactivity displayed to a stimulus by an older animal was due to lack of prior experience with it or with related stimuli. This process of learning about environmental stimuli, the process of "experiencing," was conceived of as normally high-priority behavior for the young mammal, but, most importantly, this kind of learning was endogenously motivated learning and not demanded or "directed" by the experimenter.

Noting the similarity between early environment and early malnutrition, we reasoned that malnutrition might affect cognitive processing through the same mechanism as early environmental isolation. To test this idea we performed a factorial experiment in which we raised animals under an environmentally "enriched" or an environmentally "impoverished" condition either in a well-nourished or severely malnourished state.[19] All manipulations occurred during the first 7 weeks of life, followed by 10 weeks of control diet and environmental conditions. As seen in Figure 12.4 we found a significant interaction between early environment and nutrition on later behavior. The effects of environmental isolation on locomotor behavior were exaggerated by early malnutrition, whereas environmental enrichment greatly ameliorated the effects of early malnutrition on this response. Other kinds of be-

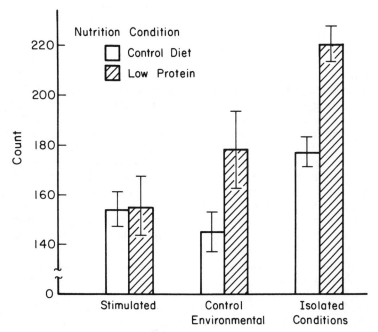

Figure 12.4. Mean and standard error of total locomotor movements per session for each treatment condition

havior showed similar effects. We interpreted these interactions between early nutrition and early environment as support for our hypothesis that malnutrition might produce its long-term effects on behavior by "functionally isolating" an animal from its environment.

It is important at this point to reflect on the ramifications of this hypothesis in terms of both data and theory. We started out with the concept that since early malnutrition caused long-term alterations in the brain, malnutrition must have damaged the brain (the hardware of the computer) and therefore left the animal with the inability to process information or learn. We could find no evidence that the ability to learn was impaired by severe malnutrition. Our alternative hypothesis was that it was the software, the programming of the computer, which was altered by malnutrition. Malnutrition prevented certain kinds of information relating to the environment from being learned. Our attention was then directed to the study of the mechanisms of "functional isolation."

The most obvious mechanisms through which malnutrition may impede the organism from learning about its environment is through a delay in skeletal-muscular growth and maturation. A delay in psychomotor development in the malnourished rat has been demonstrated by several researchers.[27, 29]

In order to observe the behavioral effect of malnutrition in the very young animal, without disturbing the animals, Massaro and I developed a photographic observation technique.[23] The major virtue of this technique was that we could collect a large number of observations for each animal without the need to have an experimenter located in the vicinity of the subjects during the period of observation. Figure 12.5 is a good example of the kinds of data collected with this technique and demonstrates quite well the effects of malnutrition on the dispersion of the litter with age. Whereas there was a very rapid dispersion of the litter of control-fed rats into the environment with development, malnourishing the dam produced a profound retardation in this behavior.

Part of this effect, we thought, was due to the delay in psychomotor development, as found by others. However, we found that malnutrition also affected the dam in such a way as to retard the delay of maternal behavior with age.

Figure 12.6 shows the percent of the total observation time the dam was observed in the presence of the litter as a function of age and malnutrition. Malnourishing the pups by malnourishing the

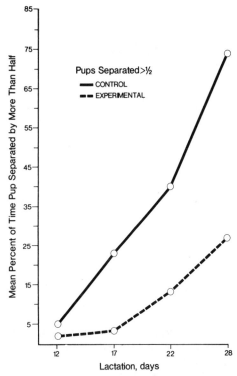

Figure 12.5. Mean percent of observations in which the pups were observed in groups of 3 or less over the period of lactation

dam increased maternal behavior as reflected by an increase in the time spent in contact with pups. How does malnutrition increase maternal behavior? Rosenblat and Lehrman presented a strong argument that one of the major determinants of maternal behavior was the size of the pup and perhaps the level of behavioral development of the pup.[25] Malnutrition obviously retards the growth of the pup. Further support for this hypothesis, however, came from our observation that the maternal behavior appeared to increase in normally fed dams nursing small-for-date pups produced naturally or because of malnutrition experienced during gestation.[21] Thus, in the very young organism both the retardation in psychomotor development and the increase in maternal behavior acted to inhibit the exploration of the environment by young malnourished organisms.

There is a third and quite important way through which mal-

David A. Levitsky

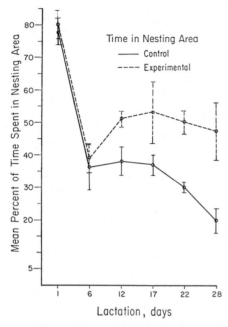

Figure 12.6. Mean percent of observations in which the dam was observed in the nesting area.

Lactation, days

nutrition isolates the young animal from its environment and that is by depressing exploratory behavior and curiosity. In our study on stimulation and malnutrition, we observed that when the weanling rats were placed in a group cage, the well-fed animals engaged in a great deal of social behavior and manipulation (play?) of the various toys scattered about the cage. A group of concurrently malnourished animals, on the other hand, spent very little time engaging in social behavior, spending instead most of their time buried inside little tunnels. Zimmerman observed similar effects in monkeys and also noted that malnourished monkeys seem to display a fear reaction to novel stimuli.[31]

We decided to look at this phenomenon in more depth using pigs.[2] After adapting the pigs to an observation room for several days we introduced a novel stimulus consisting of a large, brightly colored ball. Table 12.3 shows the results of this simple manipulation on behavior. The control animals almost immediately made contact with the object and continued to manipulate the object throughout the testing session. Pigs maintained on low-protein or low-calorie diets, however, displayed a signifi-

172

cantly greater latency to make contact and manipulated the ball to a far lesser extent than controls. We have some data to suggest that malnutrition produced the same effect in the rat. Malnutrition, then, also acted to functionally isolate the animal from its environment by depressing a naturally occurring endogenously motivated mechanism which impelled the animal to learn about its environment.

Finally, a fourth and perhaps most important mechanism through which malnutrition acts to restrict the animal from its environment may have a very fundamental effect on cognitive processing. We have previously argued that early malnutrition, or concurrent malnutrition, did not affect the rate of "directed" learning, that is, learning in situations where the attention of the organism was directed by the experimenter to the stimuli relevant for the solution of a problem.

Melzack and others have suggested, as mentioned earlier, that a basic kind of learning takes place naturally in young organisms in situations where learning is neither demanded nor directed by the experimenter and where it is without physiological motivation. This question of whether necessity is a requirement for learning to occur is a very old one in psychology. Early proponents of the argument insisted that need or drive was necessary for learning. This line of argument directed the interest of human theorists away from any serious consideration of the animal as a model for human cognitive processing, since it was clear from human experience that no physiological need was necessary for human learning to occur.

The problem of demonstrating learning without physiologically motivating animals is quite difficult, yet several experimental paradigms were created. The best known is that of tests of latent

Table 12.3. Mean latency to contact play object and total number of contacts with play objects for protein-malnourished and control pigs

	Mean latency to contact play object (min.)	Mean number of contacts with play object (counts)	P value
Controls	.638	6.49	.01
Protein malnourished	184	28.3	.001

learning.[30] To demonstrate latent learning the animal is usually placed in a maze with no food or water and left there for 4 to 10 hours. The deprived animals are then "trained" to run the maze in order to receive nutriment at the end of the maze. When the performance of these "experienced" animals is compared to the performance of a group of animals, handled in the same way, but not previously exposed to the maze, the number of errors of the experienced group in "learning" the maze is typically found to be less than the nonexperienced group. Although it still is not clear what the animals learn about the maze or the testing situation during the initial experience with the maze, it is clear that they pick up some information which is advantageous in helping them solve the problem, when learning the maze is "demanded" by the experimenter through the imposition of a physiological need.

We used the latent-learning paradigm to test the hypothesis that concurrent malnutrition might block this nondirected learning.[17] Weanling rats were used. The experiment was identical to that outlined above except that during the period of initial exposure one group was maintained on a low-protein diet (10 percent) and a comparable control group was treated the same but experienced an open field instead of the maze. The experiment was repeated twice. The first time 10 hours of initial exposure was used, followed by 4 weeks of dietary recovery before testing. The second time a 4-hour exposure was used and 8 weeks of dietary recovery was used. For testing, all animals were deprived of food for 48 hours, and four 45 mg food pellets were used as reinforcements. The total number of errors for the first five trials were used as the dependent variable. The amount of "savings" in errors for each dietary group is displayed in Table 12.4. These data suggest that the effect of experience on later learning was blocked by malnutrition.

I had thought originally that this was a clear situation in which normal well-fed animals demonstrated a kind of learning that was blocked by malnutrition. However, upon further analysis a number of problems with technique became apparent. First, the latent-learning effect occurred on the very first trial, that is, before the animal could even "know" that a reward awaited it at the end of the maze. Second, although we obtained significant interaction between the experienced and inexperienced groups in the total number of errors committed in learning the maze, there was a significant effect of malnutrition in the nonexperienced group.

Finally, as mentioned previously, it was not at all clear what was being learned during the experience in the maze.

Another paradigm and perhaps one better suited for testing our hypothesis of "nondirected" learning was the redundant-learning paradigm. In this paradigm, the animals were required to learn a problem consisting of responding correctly to a set of stimuli for a physiological reinforcement. After the animals demonstrated that they had learned the problem, they were then given additional redundant information (stimuli) for a fixed number of trials. The animals were then tested on the redundant stimuli alone in order to assess the degree of learning that occurred during the redundant phase. It should be pointed out that during the redundant phase, the animal was not required to respond to the additional information in order to solve the problem correctly.

We trained the pig to respond to a go/no-go avoidance discrimination to two auditory stimuli. To one of the auditory stimuli the pig was required to perform an avoidance response. The other auditory stimulus was safe, and no response was required. The pigs rapidly learned to discriminate between the two auditory stimuli as demonstrated by differential latency to respond to two stimuli. After performance had stabilized, two visual stimuli were paired with the auditory stimuli for 75 trials. Finally, we tested the animals by presenting the visual stimuli alone. One group of young pigs was well nourished throughout the test; another was maintained on a 6 percent protein diet. Well-nourished pigs showed significant transfer, displaying a difference in latency of 30 percent to the two visual stimuli on the first 10 trials. Pigs malnourished with the protein-poor diet showed no discrimination between the visual stimuli. We performed the necessary counterbalancing experiments to show basically the same effect if the pigs were first taught the visual discrimination, then trans-

Table 12.4. Percent savings of errors due to prior maze experience

	Experiment I*	Experiment II†
Controls	69.3	46.0
Malnourished	45.0	21.3

*Differences significant beyond .05 level.
†Differences significant beyond .01 level.

ferred to the auditory stimuli. There was no difference in original rate of conditioning.

With Goldberger, we developed a test of redundant learning in the rat using appetitive motivation.[11,17] Hungry rats were first trained to discriminate between two visual stimuli in order to receive food. After performance stabilized, the animals were given redundant stimuli for a fixed set of trials, then tested on the redundant stimuli alone. Two levels of food deprivation were used. One group was maintained at 90 percent of control body weight. The other group was maintained at 70 percent of control body weight. We found basically the same results as with the pig: the poorer the nutritional state the poorer the performance in the test for redundant learning. In the rat studies, however, we observed a significant stimulus interaction. When the redundant stimuli were salient compared to the original stimuli there was very little effect of the degree of malnutrition on redundant learning. It was only when the redundant stimuli were less salient, more subtle than the original stimuli, that the more well-nourished animals displayed superior redundant learning.

From these studies we concluded that malnutrition does not necessarily impair the ability of the rat or pig to learn, for when demanded by the experimenter these animals learn just as rapidly as well-nourished controls. Malnutrition does not seem to affect the hardware of the learning machine, but it apparently alters the program. The well-nourished mammal leaves the nest, explores its environment, and learns that it has not only to avoid pain and discomfort but also to program many other aspects about its environment, information upon which it may build more complex concepts of its world. The well-nourished, healthy, growing animal is thus programmed with a hunger to learn all about its environment, not just its essential features. This hunger to learn all about the environment is dramatically inhibited by malnutrition. The malnourished animal, apparently, responds only to those features of the environment that are of immediate biological consequence.

What is it about malnutrition that turns off the programming of nondirected, nondemanded learning behavior in the young mammal and turns on the defensive-reaction program? In our quest to find the answer to this difficult question, we have sought to find correlated changes in brain biochemistry and behavior. As is well known, early malnutrition produces profound effects in almost all chemical systems in the brain, and to find those critical changes responsible for the behavioral alteration is a formidable task. Impressed by the work of Mark Rosensweig and his colleagues who showed brain cholinesterases to be affected by environmental stimulation, we pursued the analysis of brain enzymes involved in acetylcholine metabolism. Hae Sook Im, working in our group, found that early malnutrition did indeed affect brain acetylcholine metabolism.[12, 13] Early malnutrition increased the specific activity of brain acetylcholinesterase during the period of malnutrition, and brain acetylcholinesterase remained high even after nutritional rehabilitation in both rats and pigs. This was quite an important finding to us, for it showed a change in an enzyme involved in the metabolism of a neurotransmitter, a substance known to affect behavior. These changes endured even after the period of malnutrition, as did the behavioral abnormalities.

Further work by Curtis Eckhert and our group showed that the initial rate-limiting enzyme of acetylcholine, choline acetyltransferase, was significantly depressed during and following early malnutrition.[6, 7] More importantly, concurrent environmental stimulation with malnutrition normalized the changes in these enzymes induced by malnutrition.[8, 14] This was an extremely important finding, since we had previously found that environmental stimulation during the period of malnutrition also ameliorated most of the behavioral effects of early malnutrition.[19]

It should be emphasized that these are only correlation findings. We have not proved causation. Certainly, other chemical pathways must be investigated. Other techniques and experimental paradigms must be tried to continue the attempt to find the causative links between brain chemistry and behavior. The problem is very difficult, but there is a possibility of unlocking that driving curiosity to learn in mentally impaired and malnourished children.

References

1. Altman, J. S., K. Sudarshan, G. D. Das, N. McCormick, and D. Barnes. The influence of nutrition on neural and behavioral development. III. Development of some motor, particular locomotor patterns during infancy. *Devel. Psychobiol.* 42: 97, 1971.

2. Barnes, R. H., D. A. Levitsky, W. G. Pond, and U. More. Effects of postnatal dietary protein and energy restriction on exploratory behavior in young pigs. *Devel. Psychobiol.* 9(5): 425, 1975.

3. Barnes, R. H., C. S. Neely, E. Kwong, B. A. Labadan, and S. Franková. Postnatal nutritional deprivations as determinants of adult rat behavior toward food, its consumption, and utilization. *J. Nutr.* 96: 467, 1968.

4. Collier, G. H., and R. L. Squibb. Malnutrition and the learning capacity of the chicken. In *Malnutrition, Learning, and Behavior*, N. S. Scrimshaw and J. E. Gordon, eds., M.I.T. Press, Cambridge, Mass., 1968.

5. Denenberg, V. H., and J. C. Morton. Infantile stimulation, prepubertal sexual-social interaction and emotionality. *Anim. Behav.* 12: 11, 1964.

6. Eckhert, C. D., R. H. Barnes, and D. A. Levitsky. The effect of protein energy undernutrition induced during the period of suckling on cholinergic enzyme activity in the rat brainstem. *Brain Res.* 101: 372, 1976.

7. Eckhert, C. D., R. H. Barnes, and D. A. Levitsky. Regional changes in rat brain choline acetyltransferase and acetylcholinesterase activity resulting from undernutrition imposed during different periods of development. *J. Neurochem.* 27: 277, 1976.

8. Eckhert, C. D., D. A. Levitsky, and R. H. Barnes. Postnatal stimulation: The effects on cholinergic enzyme activity in undernourished rats. *Proc. Soc. Exp. Biol. Med.* 149: 860, 1975.

9. Franková, S., and R. H. Barnes. Influence of malnutrition in early life on exploratory behavior of rats. *J. Nutr.* 96: 477, 1968.

10. Geber, M., and R. F. Dean. Psychological changes accompanying kwashiorkor. *Courrier* 6: 3, 1956.

11. Goldberger, L. I. Role of motivation and cue salience in incidental learning in the rat. Unpublished Ph.D. Thesis, Cornell University, 1976.

12. Im, H. S., R. H. Barnes, and D. A. Levitsky. Postnatal malnutrition and brain cholinesterase in rats. *Nature* (London) 233: 269, 1971.

13. Im, H. S., R. H. Barnes, D. A. Levitsky, and W. G. Pond. Postnatal malnutrition and regional cholinesterase activities in brain of pigs. *Brain Res.* 63: 461, 1973.

14. Im, H. S., R. H. Barnes, and D. A. Levitsky. Effect of early protein-energy malnutrition and environmental changes on cholinesterase activity of brain and adrenal glands of rats. *J. Nutr.* 106: 342, 1976.

15. Lashley, K. S. *Brain Mechanisms and Intelligence.* University of Chicago Press, Chicago, 1929.

16. Levine, S. The effects of differential stimulation on emotionality at weaning. *Canad. J. Psychol.* 13: 243, 1959.

17. Levitsky, D. A. Malnutrition and animal models of cognitive development. Proc. Kittay Scientific Foundation, in *Nutrition and Mental Functions*, George Serban, ed., Plenum Press, New York, 1975.

18. Levitsky, D. A., and R. H. Barnes. Effect of early malnutrition on the reaction of adult rats to aversive stimuli. *Nature* 225: 468, 1970.

19. Levitsky, D. A., and R. H. Barnes. Nutritional and environmental interactions in behavioral development of the rat: Long-term effects. *Science* 176: 68, 1972.

20. Levitsky, D., and R. H. Barnes. Malnutrition and animal behavior. In *Nutrition, Development, and Social Behavior*, D. J. Kallen, ed., U.S. DHEW, Publ. No. (NIH) #73-242, Washington, D.C., 1973.

21. Levitsky, D. A., T. F. Massaro, and R. H. Barnes. Maternal malnutrition and the neonatal environment. *Fed. Proc.* 34(7): 1583, 1975.

22. Marx, M. H. Infantile deprivation and adult behavior in the rat. Retention of increased rate of eating. *J. Comp. Physiol. Psychol.* 45: 43, 1952.

23. Massaro, T. F., D. A. Levitsky, and R. H. Barnes. Protein malnutrition in the rat: Its effect on maternal behavior and pup development. *Devel. Psychobiol.* 7: 551, 1974.

24. Melzack, R. Effects of early experience on behavior: Experimental and conceptual considerations. In *Disorders of Perception*, P. H. Hoch and J. Zubin, eds., Gruen and Stratten, New York, 1965.

25. Rosenblat, J. S., and D. S. Lehrman. Maternal behavior in the laboratory rat. In *Maternal Behavior in Mammals*, H. L. Rheingold, ed., Wiley, New York, 1963, p. 8–56.

26. Scrimshaw, N. S., and J. E. Gordon, eds., *Malnutrition, Learning, and Behavior*, M.I.T. Press, Cambridge, Mass., 1968.

27. Simonson, M., R. W. Sherwin, J. K. Anilane, W. Y. Yu, and B. F. Chow. Neuromotor development in progeny of underfed mother rats. *J. Nutr.* 98: 18, 1968.

28. Smart, J. L. Activity and exploratory behavior of adult offspring of undernourished mother rats. *Devel. Psychobiol.* 7: 315, 1974.

29. Smart, J. L., and J. Dobbing. Vulnerability of developing brain. VI. Relative effects of foetal and early postnatal undernutrition on reflex ontogeny and development of behavior in the rat. *Brain Res.* 33: 304, 1971.

30. Tolman, E. C., and C. H. Honzig. Introduction and removal of reward, and maze performance in rats. *Univ. Calif. Publication, Psychol.* 4: 257, 1930.

31. Zimmermann, R. R., D. A. Strobel, and D. Maguire. Neophobic reactions in protein malnourished infant monkeys. *Proc. 78th Annual Conv. APA* 6: 197, 1970.

James L. Smart **13**

Discussion

I wish to share with you some questions that have worried me about the field of early undernutrition and behavior over the last few years. My first concern is with the inconsistency of the results in the animal literature. Let me emphasize this: there are consistencies, and I think that there are more consistencies than Seymour Levine would have us believe. But there certainly are inconsistencies as well. One research group reports an effect of early undernutrition; yet when the experiment is repeated, or apparently repeated, in another laboratory, no effect is found.

One pretty obvious possible source of these differences is genotype X early-treatment interaction. By this I mean that animals of different genotype, different in their genetic constitution, may respond differently to the same environmental treatment. At long last, this has been investigated as a subject in its own right. I refer here to the recent work of Randt and Blizard at the New York University Medical Center.[3] This is also being investigated in Rome by Alberto Oliverio. The approach should have been made some time ago, and I am delighted to see it happening now.

Most of us dismiss the possibility of investigating one particular kind of genotype X early-treatment interaction every time we do an experiment. We discard the female members of the litter, usually at weaning, and we decide to study only the male animals. The reason is that we have read that the effects of early undernutrition on body growth are less in females[4] or are perhaps not apparent at all in their behavior.[1,2] I would suggest that the evidence for this latter statement is not very substantial. It is based on intact females, that is on females with functional ovaries, with an estrous cycle that is effectively a built-in source of variance for many aspects of behavior. This makes it much more difficult to obtain statistically significant effects of early treatment.

There have been two early undernutrition studies of ovariectomized female rats. One of these was performed by Slob and his colleagues in Rotterdam,[7] where they investigated the long-term activity, measured automatically over several days, of previously undernourished ovariectomized females. These females were significantly more active than ovariectomized controls that had been well fed in early life. The other study was conducted by Whatson et al.,[8] who were examining the social behavior of previously undernourished rats, and had already found differences in male rats as a result of early undernutrition. They decided to extend the investigation to female rats. The experimental females were growth-retarded during both gestation and the suckling period by underfeeding their mothers, and were then allowed a lengthy period of nutritional rehabilitation, during which time they had free access to a good-quality diet. All females were ovariectomized in adulthood some 4 weeks before observation. Eleven pairs of rats were observed, each comprising one control and one previously undernourished female. These same pairs were observed 10 minutes a day on 8 days. The previously undernourished females performed significantly more allogrooming and crawl-under responses than their control partners (Figure 13.1). They were almost always more socially responsive. The important point is that these differences between ovariectomized females were very similar to those that had been observed between males.[9]

I am making a plea here for further study of genotype X early-treatment interaction. First, let us investigate this variable in its own right. Second, let us use females as well as males; and here, to reduce variance, it may be useful to ovariectomize the females. Third, let us use different species. A review of the literature on early undernutrition reveals that about 80 percent of the papers are on rats. There are a number now on mice, a few from Cornell on pigs, and reports are beginning to trickle through of studies with primates. Another species is introduced in Chapter 10, above, where Simonson describes her investigation of malnourished cats. Let us continue to diversify, and then any extrapolations or generalizations that we make from animals to human beings will be that much better substantiated.

My next concern is a difficult one to resolve. The correspondence between the results of animal and human studies is not always good. First, let us take what might loosely be called learning ability. If we review the literature on this for rats, for instance,

James L. Smart

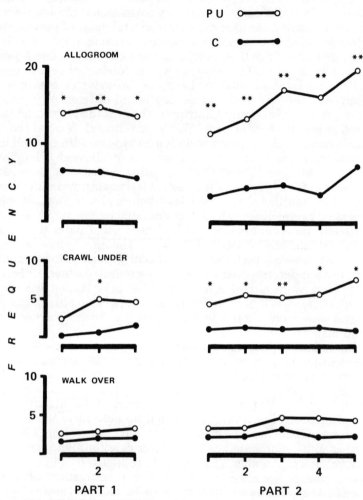

Figure 13.1. Mean frequencies of 3 social responses performed by ovariectomized female control (C) and previously undernourished (PU) rats during 8 daily test sessions, each of 10 minutes duration. Ten days elapsed between parts 1 and 2 of the observation period. All 11 C and 11 PU rats had been ovariectomized at least 4 weeks before testing. (According to Wilcoxon matched-pairs signed-ranks test, p < 0.05;* p < 0.01.**)

we emerge confused. The results are equivocal. It certainly cannot be said that there is any consistent effect of early undernutrition on learning ability. But if we review the literature on previously malnourished children, we find that their IQ's are almost always down a few points. This is perplexing.

Second, let us consider social behavior. Our previously undernourished male rats are more aggressive to one another than are control animals; and, in general, both males and females are more socially responsive. This is borne out in the work of Levitsky and Barnes at Cornell and Fraňková in Prague. If we look at the literature on man, however, the little existing evidence is in marked contrast. Two quotations from the same study of previously malnourished Jamaican children illustrate my point. The first quotation[5] refers to the children's behavior in school (I should explain that the term "index" means previously malnourished in this quotation): "The composite picture that emerges of the index boys' behavior is that of a passive, quiet and withdrawn child rather than one who is aggressive and tends to act out." The information in the second quotation[6] is based on interviews with the boys' parents: "The index boys are described more frequently as . . . withdrawn, solitary or unsociable," and "less often than their classmates as aggressive, stubborn or disobedient." Nothing, as far as I can see, could be more diametrically opposed to the results that several of us have obtained for rats.

These inconsistencies are a source of some worry to me. I can explain them away to myself, as I feel I must from time to time, but I confess that I am not fully satisfied with my explanations. I should be interested to find out how others react to these sorts of difficulty.

Finally, I should like to comment on Levitsky's work (Chapter 12, above). I found the elegant experiments on redundant learning especially interesting, and I can well appreciate the temptation to extrapolate their results far beyond the context of those particular experiments. I think that we should be clear that they were carried out with rats which were currently in a state of nutritional deprivation, and that this is rather different from the usual early undernutrition paradigm in which the animals are tested several weeks or even months after the period of nutritional privation. Hence great caution ought to be exercised in extrapolating their results to previously malnourished animals or to human beings.

The sort of experiment which I should now like to see made

would have the following among its characteristics: animals would be given the opportunity for redundant learning during a period of early life undernutrition; much later, after several weeks of nutritional "rehabilitation," they would be tested for evidence of this learning. Even if deficiencies of redundant learning were demonstrated in such an experiment, the difficult question still remains: Does it really matter that this "hunger to learn" is temporarily damped down? Presumably it does, if there are age-specific, critical periods for learning certain things. If not, then it may be relatively unimportant.

References

1. Barnes, R. H., S. R. Cunnold, R. R. Zimmermann, H. Simmons, R. B. MacLeod, and L. Krook. Influence of nutritional deprivations in early life on learning behavior of rats as measured by performance in a water maze. *J. Nutr.* 89: 399, 1966.

2. Barnes, R. H., A. U. Moore, I. M. Reid, and W. G. Pond. Learning behavior following nutritional deprivations in early life. *J. Am. Dietet. Assn.* 51: 34, 1967.

3. Blizard, D. A., and C. T. Randt. Genotype interaction with undernutrition and external environment in early life. *Nature* (London) 251: 705, 1974.

4. Kennedy, G. C. The development with age of hypothalamic restraint upon the appetite of the rat. *J. Endocri.* 16: 9, 1955.

5. Richardson, S. A., H. G. Birch, E. Grabie, and K. Yoder. The behavior of children in school who were severely malnourished in the first two years of life. *J. Health Soc. Behav.* 13: 276, 1972.

6. Richardson, S. A., H. G. Birch, and C. Ragbeer. The behavior of children at home who were severely malnourished in the first two years of life. *J. Biosoc. Sci.* 7: 255, 1975.

7. Slob, A. K., C. E. Snow, and E. de Natris-Mathot. Absence of behavioral deficits following neonatal undernutrition in the rat. *Devel. Psychobiol.* 6: 177, 1973.

8. Whatson, T. S., J. L. Smart, and J. Dobbing. Social interactions among adult male rats after early undernutrition. *Brit. J. Nutr.* 32: 413, 1974.

9. Whatson, T. S., J. L. Smart, and J. Dobbing. Undernutrition in early life: Lasting effects on activity and social behavior of male and female rats. *Devel. Psychobiol.* 9: 529, 1976.

Victor H. Denenberg **14**

Discussion

I know little about malnutrition, but I have spent about 20 years doing research in developmental psychobiology, and the perspective that I bring to my comments is that of a person who has been studying early experiences and developmental processes for many years.

Thus, if I were going to do research in the area of malnutrition and behavior, I would ask the following question: What are the long-term effects of malnutrition? If we wish to answer that question by use of an animal model—and we will let the rat be our experimental subject—we have certain necessary conditions which must be met. The first condition is that *there must be a sufficient number of litters per treatment group.* The exact number is hard to specify unless one knows some of the statistical characteristics of one's variable. As a rough rule of thumb somewhere between 4 and 12 litters would be a reasonable place to start as we begin the design of the experiment.

The second necessary condition is that *the data must be analyzed by the proper statistical design.* Littermates are *not* independent observations. They are correlated because of genetic heritage, and by common intrauterine and postnatal environmental conditions. There are several ways to control for this. One way is to use only one subject per litter. This is the procedure that Simonson has used in her research. Another approach is to use the litter mean as a single score. A third way is to use all the individuals of the litter. The third suggestion, however, is based upon the assumption that all the animals in the study are independent observations, and it is necessary to statistically justify this assumption, since—as noted above—littermates tend to be correlated. The necessary statistical procedure is to perform an analysis of variance to determine whether "mean square between litters" is statistically larger than "mean square within litters." If the mean square between litters is larger, then it is not permissible to use the individual subject as the unit for statistical analysis, and the litter mean must be used instead. For a detailed discussion of this topic see the papers by Abbey and Howard[1] and Denenberg.[4] *We must also have a control for the effects of maternal behavior.* Malnutrition imposed during lactation profoundly affects the behavior of the dam. Thus, even if significant behavioral effects of lactational malnutrition are observed, it is impossible to determine whether the effects are caused by the malnutrition, per se, or by the altered maternal behavior.

How can we control for the effects of maternal behavior? One procedure is to cross-foster at birth. This is a valid way to assess the effects of *prenatal* malnutrition. If one is concerned with *postnatal* malnutrition, then the use of a rat-aunt preparation—a procedure we developed[6]—can be used. This is the technique that Fraňková has employed. If long-term effects can be demonstrated with such controls, this will make it more reasonable to conclude that early malnutrition may be causally involved.

I must emphasize that it is necessary that these minimal conditions of experimental design be met in order to answer any question as to the long-term effects of early malnutrition. Unfortunately, when I read the literature, I find very few studies that meet all of these criteria. There is no doubt but that an enormous number of changes take place in a variety of physiological, endocrinological, biochemical, and behavioral systems *during the time that the animal is malnourished.* The critical question, however, is whether there are any lasting effects observable after nutritional rehabilitation.

If I were to apply rigorously the criteria listed above, I would restrict myself to a few comments on Simonson's papers, because the work by Levitsky, Fraňková, and Barnes do not satisfy these criteria. However, I am not stopping here for several reasons: (1) even though these criteria are not all satisfied, several theoretical concepts have been put forth which should be discussed; (2) some of the data might be interesting even though the experimental design is insufficient; (3) this is a very emotional area, and there are researchers who are in essence saying, "Don't bother me with facts; I am a firm believer in what I believe"; and (4) neither journal editors nor granting agencies apparently consider these criteria in the publication of papers or the awarding of money. (I do not mean to imply that only Levitsky, Barnes, and Fraňková have weaknesses in their experimental procedures and statistical analyses. Most of the research papers I have read are equally weak, and some of them are just terrible.)

A concept that Winick noted (Chapter 9, above) and that has been mentioned several times is the one put forth by Levitsky and Barnes on "functional isolation." The concept, I think, is well described by a quotation from an article by Massaro, Levitsky, and Barnes.[10]

The results of the present study support the hypothesis that early malnutrition may produce its long-lasting effects on adult behavior by functionally isolating the organism from its environment during the period of malnutrition. The most impressive feature of the normal development of pup behavior is the increase in behavior associated with environmental exploration. This process is severely altered in the malnourished pup. Feeding the dam a low-protein diet not only affects the physiological growth of the pup but produces a whole set of interactive behaviors between the pup and the dam, the functional consequence of which is a decrease in exploration of the environment by the pup.

The concept is interesting. I firmly believe in one part of the concept, namely that the interaction of the mother with her pups is one of the major determinants of the pups' later behavior. We have shown that the mother's behavior affects behavioral, physical, and physiological processes of her offspring or foster offspring.[3, 5, 7, 9, 11]

Thus, the principle that mother-pup interactions affect later pup performance rests upon a sound data base. However, the broader concept of functional isolation, as put forth in the Massaro, Levitsky, and Barnes paper, does not rest upon a firm data base. Unfortunately, the analyses of variance in that paper are all in error. In examining those analyses, I expect that probably one-half to two-thirds of the statistics would be verified when the proper analyses are done, but not all of them. I am quite certain of that. Therefore, part of the data base for the concept of functional isolation is not there, and that raises the serious issue of the validity of the concept.

Another challenge to the notion of functional isolation derives from the concept of "risk." that is, the animal that is functionally isolated is at risk for something. Yet we do not find much evidence that the 3 weeks of presumed maladaptive interaction between the mother and the pups brings about any major harm. The data are as follows: Barnes et al. in 1966 studied Y-maze perfor-

187

mance of animals that had been on deprivation diets during early development.[2] They found that rats deprived prenatally and prior to weaning did not differ from controls. They did get an effect in another group that also had postweaning deprivation experience, but the important point is that the prenatal and preweaning experience of malnutrition had no measurable behavioral effect. Also, in that paper, it was reported that the females were not affected. It is difficult to understand why the concept of functional isolation should be chauvanistic with respect to sex, but possibly that is so.

Fraňková and Barnes found no effect upon the latency to respond to the conditioned stimulus, which was the best measure they had of learning.[8] There was an effect upon the measure of time spent upon the test screen. However, this was only for the group that received deprivation conditions after weaning, not before weaning. From my reading in the literature from the Cornell group, there is certainly very little evidence that preweaning malnutrition in combination with prenatal malnutrition has any interesting or important effects upon adult behavior. If an effect cannot be determined, then the concept of functional isolation does not seem to be applicable.

This is not to say that there are no effects of early malnutrition. In terms of the criteria I have listed here, the papers by Simonson and her group are acceptable: they had an adequate number of litters per treatment condition; they typically sampled one animal per litter; and they cross-fostered 24 hours after birth to normal mothers, thus allowing for rehabilitation. They reported effects of malnutrition upon emotional responses, open-field performance, and upon the development of neuromotor acts. They have been properly cautious in their interpretations, except that Simonson made a statement about a learning process which I would challenge. I agree instead with Levitsky that it is very difficult to show a difference in learning. One can show differences in performance using a learning apparatus, but that is quite different from saying that the process of learning is itself affected.

In conclusion, there are several statements I want to make.

1. There is an almost desperate need for proper experimental designs in this area.

2. There definitely is evidence that prenatal treatment will affect some behavioral processes, and the Simonson data are the best that I have seen on this. However, since the Cornell group

usually does not find effects, their failure suggests that the effects may be strain specific, or restricted by local conditions.

3. I do not know of any evidence as yet of a permanent learning deficit. There is evidence for motivational deficit and other performance measures, but not of learning or cognitive deficits.

4. I am quite certain that the locus of effect is probably as much involved in the mother-pup interactin as it is with the nutritional level.

5. I feel that interventions other than food will have rehabilitating effects. The Levitsky and Barnes procedure of intervening with enriched environmental conditions and by handling, and the technique that Fraňková used of introducing the rat aunt show the kinds of environmental interactions that appear to have interesting and apparently "beneficial" effects, even though the designs are ones I am willing to challenge.

6. Finally, to find the effects of malnutrition, other kinds of designs must be used. To know how malnutrition interacts with peers, with the environment, with the mother, other types of experiments are called for. I think we are at the point now where we can improve, and need to improve, the sophistication of our experimental designs to answer some of the interesting questions that have been raised.

References

1. Abbey, H., and E. Howard. Statistical procedures in developmental studies on species with multiple offspring. *Devel. Psychobiol.* 6: 329, 1973.

2. Barnes, R. H., S. R. Cunnold, R. R. Zimmermann, H. Simmons, R. B. MacLeod, and L. Krook. Influence of nutritional deprivations in early life on learning behavior of rats as measured by performance in a water maze. *J. Nutr.* 89: 399, 1966.

3. Denenberg, V. H. The mother as motivator. In *Nebraska Symposium on Motivation*, W. J. Arnold and M. M. Page, eds., University of Nebraska Press, Lincoln, Nebr., 1970, p. 69–93.

4. Denenberg, V. H. Assessing the effects of early experience. In *Methods in Psychobiology*, III, R. D. Myers, ed., Academic Press, New York, 1977.

5. Denenberg, V. H., W. R. Holloway, and M. J. Dollinger. Weight gain as a consequence of maternal behavior in the rat. *Behav. Biol.* 17: 51, 1976.

6. Denenberg, V. H., K. M. Rosenberg, R. Paschke, and M. X. Zarrow. Mice reared with rat aunts: Effects on plasma corticosterone and open field activity. *Nature* 221, 73, 1969.

7. Dollinger, M. J., W. R. Holloway, and V. H. Denenberg. An interactive model determining body weight in the newborn rat. Paper presented at Annual Meet. Internat. Soc. Devel. Psychobiol., 31 Oct.–2 Nov., 1975.

8. Fraňková, S., and R. H. Barnes. Effect of malnutrition in early life on avoidance conditioning and behavior of adult rats. *J. Nutr.* 96: 485, 1968.

9. Holloway, W. R., M. J. Dollinger, and V. H. Denenberg. Factors affecting mother-pup interaction in the rat. Paper presented at Annual Meet. Internat. Soc. Devel. Psychobiol., 31 Oct.–2 Nov., 1975.

10. Massaro, T. F., D. A. Levitsky, and R. H. Barnes. Protein malnutrition in the rat: Its effects on maternal behavior and pup development. *Devel. Psychobiol.* 7: 551, 1974.

11. Ottinger, D. R., V. H. Denenberg, and M. W. Stephens. Maternal emotionality, multiple mothering, and emotionality in maturity. *J. Comp. Physiol. Psychol.* 56: 313, 1963.

PART IV

MALNUTRITION AND
PRIMATE BEHAVIOR

Behavior and Malnutrition in Nonhuman Primates

Early Monkey Studies

Preliminary research was established at the Montana Primate Laboratory to examine the effects of diets severely restricted in protein content on the social development of four 1-year-old rhesus monkeys. Although the dietary restrictions were severe (3.5 percent protein by weight or 3.3 percent calories), the feed was a complete protein (casein). Control animals were provided a diet containing 25 percent protein but isocaloric with respect to the experimental diet. These purified diets were found easy to mix and were highly palatable.

The early months of dietary restriction passed with some apprehension. There were few studies to provide information on whether monkeys could survive on the restricted diets, and they were watched carefully for signs that they might perish without protein supplementation.

The protein-deficient diets produced a marked effect on weight gain. The malnourished monkeys gained only 15 percent over a two-year period, whereas controls tripled their weight over the same period. Significantly lowered total protein, albumin, and albumin/globulin ratios were found in the blood serum of the malnourished animals;[8] their hair became brittle, and within a few months they showed considerable denudement; the malnourished animals nonetheless appeared healthy and active. Furthermore, they did not develop edema.

In comparison, swine have been reported to develop a kwashiorkorlike syndrome, including edema, when fed high-fat diets containing very small quantities of protein.[21,22] On the other hand, young rhesus monkeys subjected to postnatal protein restrictions did not show the classical signs of clinical kwashior-

David Strobel

kor.[12,20] The only reliable means for producing all essential features of kwashiorkor in monkeys reportedly involved a tube-feeding technique.[3,23] It is possible that our pilot animals did not develop edema because they limited their caloric intake, consuming less food than the controls. Interestingly, when daily food consumption was computed with regard to body weight, this proportion was found to be equivalent for both experimental and control subjects.

Tests for discrimination learning, manipulation, and social behavior were conducted to explore a variety of behavioral conditions that might be affected by the protein malnutrition.[37] Within a month following the onset of protein restriction, alterations were found in curiosity, manipulation, and social behavior. The protein-malnourished monkeys, however, were not found inferior to controls on operant conditioning or discrimination learning tasks. Contrariwise, the low-protein subjects were clearly superior to well-fed monkeys after an initial training experience in the particular test apparatus.

Additional Groups

The successful rearing of 1-year-old monkeys on protein-deficient diets provided the incentive to explore additional groups of animals. Research at this time was very much influenced by the notion that relatively permanent or long-term behavioral and physiological changes would occur with dietary restrictions during the period of greatest brain growth. This age variable is often stated as a "critical period" hypothesis.[4,33] Unfortunately, the high mortality rates among severely undernourished newborn monkeys reported by Kerr and Waisman[12] were prohibitive for our small laboratory. It was decided, therefore, to examine longer-term, postweaning forms of malnutrition.

The standard procedure was to separate the baby monkeys from their mothers at day 90 of age and to house them individually in wire cages. The infants were fed a Prosoybee formula until they were weaned to a solid food diet containing 25 percent protein. The low-protein diets (3.5 percent casein by weight) were introduced to half the population of animals (total n = 6) at either day 120 or day 210 of age.

A significant decline in blood serum total protein and weight gain were recorded within the first month on the low-protein diets.[8] A single 1.5-year-old monkey developed symptoms of

194

kwashiorkor, including "flaky-paint rash" on the body and extremities, "moist groin rash" of the genitals, brittle depigmented and sparse hair, hypoalbuminemia and hypoproteinemia, and edema of the face and extremities. This animal subsequently died of lobar pneumonia. However, it was patently clear that this was an unusual case. The other protein-deprived animals readily adapted to the restriction and even began to gain weight after three years on the diet.

Immediately following weaning, the monkeys were adapted to a Wisconsin General Test Apparatus (WGTA) to prepare them for discrimination and other learning tasks. The high- and low-protein monkeys did not differ significantly in delayed response, six-trial-learning set, reversal learning, or long-term retention tests. It was necessary to mildly deprive the high-protein monkeys throughout the test periods because of motivational differences between the malnourished animals and the controls. It might be suggested that the detection of differences in learning capacity was masked by the confounding effects of motivational differences when food was offered as a reward for instrumental responses. To counter this argument, learning experiments were conducted using aversive reinforcers. However, the low-protein monkeys were found to have lower thresholds for response to electric shock.[31] Furthermore, the malnourished animals exhibited maladaptive behaviors in response to the shock, often self-clutching and falling into a fetal position without making a single escape response. These competing behaviors, therefore, made it impossible to investigate complex learning motivated by electrical shock.

A new apparatus was designed to test the monkeys on an aversive task that did not require electrical shock. The subjects received a blast of compressed air if an incorrect response was made in a two-choice discrimination situation. The apparatus was adapted to the WGTA to investigate the development of learning set. Again, no significant differences in performance were found between the malnourished monkeys and the well-fed controls. All animals showed adequate formation of learning set.[26]

At this point deficiencies in learning ability of any kind in the groups of malnourished monkeys were not found. Casual observation, however, indicated that the low-protein subjects were more tense and agitated than the controls, particularly in response to novel situations or new testing personnel. In addition, there was evidence that the malnourished monkeys were less interested in manipulating puzzles or pulling chains than controls when the only extrinsic reinforcement available was the manipulation itself.[1,27]

Specific tests were conducted to measure the monkeys' reaction to novelty. When bright and shiny objects were attached to chains suspended in the home cage, the high-protein monkeys significantly increased their chain-pulling rates. In contrast, there was an almost total suppression of chain-pulling exhibited by the experimental subjects. In addition, the malnourished animals avoided responding to a novel object in the WGTA when it was paired with a familiar stimulus. This occurred even when the familiar object of the pair was previously experienced by the subject as a negative stimulus (always nonrewarded). Normal monkeys, in comparison, tended to approach the novel object even when it was paired with a familiar object that had been consistently reinforced.[38] Finally, novel objects were found to disrupt an ongoing instrumental response and to suppress that response until the objects became familiar through experience.[35]

A new tack was taken in a continued search for tasks that might differentiate the learning performances of malnourished groups from controls. The original response to the failure to find these differences centered on the possibility that the diets produced subtle changes in learning performance that remained undetected by our early, "crude" behavioral designs. Another possibility was that the wrong questions were being asked. Suppose there were no real differences between the diet groups in the capacity to learn, but that other nonassociative variables could be used to differentiate the behavioral performances of animals? For example, the animals must be able to look for and find the discriminative cue or cues before they can respond successfully in a discrimination problem. The ability to select the stimulus dimension that is rewarded and localize the cue that indicates a correct response is often termed the process of attention. Klein et al.[13] found that children with a history of malnutrition did not necessarily differ on simple discrimination learning tasks, per se, but were inferior to normal controls on tasks that placed increasing demands upon attentional processes.

Stimuli were constructed that minimized or maximized the demands placed on attentional mechanisms in discrimination reversal problems.[39] The reversal paradigm forced the subjects to give up a previously successful discriminative cue that denoted the location of reward and required a search for new discriminative cues. Increased demands on attentional mechanisms were manipulated by making the new discriminative cues increasingly more difficult to locate. As a consequence, the low-protein monkeys were found significantly inferior to controls on all but the least difficult reversal problems. While food rewards were used in this study, the high-protein monkeys were mildly food deprived and were provided with high-incentive food rewards. In this manner the original learning performances of all groups were equated before the critical tests on reversal problems. This was the first learning task we found that successfully differentiated malnourished monkeys from their well-fed peers. Subsequent tasks that spatially (pattern strings), or temporally (conditional learning) separated the cue from the locus of the response were also successful in differentiating the performance of the groups.[35] The ability of malnourished animals to transfer responses to a hidden or embedded figure was also found to be greatly impaired. In sum, it is evident that if attentional mechanisms were necessary for the performance of the problems we presented, then these mechanisms appeared disrupted by the nutrition variable. The question remains whether this is the direct or indirect effect of the nutritional manipulation.

The monkeys were tested in a social playroom in their respective groups at least twice a week over a two-year period.[36] Two purposes were served by these tests. First, a minimum of social contact with peers was necessary to prevent young monkeys from developing abnormal behavior patterns found to result from social restrictions.[25] Second, if learning ability, motiviation, or perception were in any way affected by the variable of malnutrition, differences would be expected in the social situation. The complex rules governing social intercourse are largely acquired through extended experience with adults and peers. Because these experiences normally involve rapid and often novel changes in the stimulus environment, multiple discriminations, concept learning, and memory mechanisms are essential for these interactions.

Systematic observations revealed that the protein-malnourished animals differed significantly from control groups in their patterns of social contact. The low-protein monkeys showed less sexual behavior, play behavior, and fewer grooming responses.

197

They spent more time apart than the high-protein animals, and when they did make social contact with a conspecific, the meeting was typified by aggression and brutality. Hyperaggression and reduced social contacts are also typical patterns found in rhesus monkeys reared in partial social isolation.[10, 16, 17, 25]

It was noticed in the laboratory that over the two-year period of testing, the malnourished monkeys increasingly showed a tendency to avoid each other by sitting apart and withdrawing when approached. It was supposed that by maintaining social distance, the low-protein subjects avoided the aversive consequences resulting from contact. Biweekly opportunities for socialization, therefore, were of little assistance to the malnourished monkeys. They appeared trapped in a vicious circle: by not interacting when provided the opportunity, they engaged in self-inflicted separation, thus producing functional isolation and extending the conditions of the home-cage separation.

Following these early social observations, it was speculated that malnutrition interfered with normal social development of the monkey in a manner analagous to that produced by more direct forms of social isolation. Levitsky and Barnes[14] suggested that early malnutrition in rodents and swine might alter the animal's responsivity to stress through mechanisms probably related to insufficiency of environmental stimulation. Furthermore, these authors have provided evidence from rat studies that the combination of malnutrition and environmental restriction produced a significant interaction that severely debilitated the developing organism.

Following Barnes's advice we took the next obvious step in the development of our research. An experiment was designed to more directly examine the possible interactive effects of protein malnutrition and environmental rearing conditions.

Malnutrition and Early Social Experience

Six groups of at least four monkeys each were formed. The animals were all reared by their mothers until they were separated at day 90 of age. Half of the animals were placed on the experimental diets (3.5 percent protein) at day 120 of age, and the remaining animals were maintained on the control diets (25 percent protein). Three rearing conditions were established in each diet group: (ISO) partial isolates that were reared in separate living cages without peer-peer social contact for the first year of life;

(DSE) that were social tested in the playroom beginning at day 120 of age for 3 to 5 days a week; (ENR) that were housed together in large group cages and were social tested in the playroom after their first year of life.

Analysis of social observations recorded over a 12-month period during the second year of life have been presented in detail elsewhere.[35] There were a number of major trends, however, worth mentioning. The diet groups, for example, were distinguishable in the incidence and duration of active social contacts. The protein-malnourished groups were found to be significantly more aggressive in their social contacts than controls. The low-protein (ISO) monkeys showed the most agonistic behavior, and the high-protein group (ENR) the least number of such encounters. Providing some weekly socialization during the first year of life, however, significantly helped the protein-malnourished (DSE) monkeys to reduce the incidence of aggression. Conversely, the high-protein monkeys engaged in significantly more play behaviors than the malnourished animals, with the (ENR) animals showing more approach-play than the (DSE) or (ISO) groups. The low-protein monkeys spent most of their time oriented toward inanimate objects, or displayed nonsocial behaviors involving sitting, pacing without visible direction, or self-oriented responses.

The diets had no measurable effect on the frequency or duration of tactual contact, including mutual clinging or clutching. However, there were significant differences found in contacts made by animals of different rearing conditions. Monkeys that lived together as a group spent significantly more time in peaceful physical contact with each other than did groups reared apart. There were qualitative differences in the type of tactual contact. In the low-protein (ENR) group, this contact was classified as infantile, typically involving clinging or clutching. In comparison, the high-protein (ENR) monkeys engaged in significantly more mature contacts than the other groups, involving touching, body exploration, and grooming responses.

Other relationships between the development of social behavior in the monkey and dietary factors and social rearing experiences were highly complex. Some behaviors appeared to be altered more by diets, while others appeared under the control of social rearing variables. In general, the social behavior of the high-protein (ENR) monkeys more closely approximated the patterns described for normally developing monkeys under simulated "optimal" ecological conditions.[25] The low-protein (ISO) animals showed behavior patterns most deviate from this ideal, while the other groups showed responses between these two extremes.

It was hypothesized that the hyperaggression observed in the malnourished monkeys might be related to the disrupted development of dominance roles. A series of studies were established to quantify the stability of the social organizations.[30, 31, 32] The monkeys were measured for dominance/aggressive and subordinate/submissive interactions in the playroom using a system developed by Locke, Locke, Morgan, and Zimmermann.[15] In another test, all combinations of animal pairings competed for food rewards in a WGTA or in parallel sets of cages. Finally, dominance status was measured by forcing the monkeys to compete for escape or avoidance of electrical shock.

The protein-malnourished animals were found to be significantly inferior to the larger well-nourished control monkeys when ranked by social interactive measures. On the other hand, the low-protein subjects were highly successful in out-competing the high-protein animals when food became the incentive for competition. When shock was used as the incentive to exert dominance, the larger well-fed controls were found to be significantly more dominant. It would appear then that an enhanced motivation for food induced the protein-deficient monkeys to overcome their typical subordinate reactions to high-protein animals.

When the animals reached four years of age they were retested in the social playroom. It was hypothesized earlier[36] that malnourished animals physically isolated themselves when placed in a social situation. The experimenters therefore recorded the spatial location of each animal in the social room every five minutes as well as measures of frequencies and durations of social and object oriented categories of behavior. The location was transcribed as a three-digit code and computer analyzed. The results of 280 observations are summarized in Table 15.1.

The high-protein (ENR) monkeys maintained the closest proximity during the observation periods, while the low-protein (ISO) subjects showed the greatest spatial disparity. These results are consistent with the concurrent observation that the malnourished animals engaged in fewer social contacts and approach-play activities than controls. The partial-isolate groups spent more than half their social contact time engaged in agonistic behaviors (low-protein [ISO] = 62.6 percent; high-protein [ISO] = 51.8 percent).

Table 15.1. Average proximity (in centimeters) of animals in social playroom

	Rearing condition	
Diet conditions	Partial isolate	Social enriched
Low protein	176.4	141.4
High protein	150.1	127.9

In comparison, the low-protein and high-protein socially enriched animals had only 18.5 percent and 11.1 percent of their social contact time classified as agonistic, respectively.

Further, specialized categories of behavior were observed during the social tests. These behaviors included behaviors described as being typical of immature monkeys,[24] or "abnormal" responses which have been described in rhesus monkeys raised under various degrees of isolation during early development.[10, 11, 16, 19, 28, 29]

Table 15.2 indicates that the low-protein (ISO) monkeys showed the highest incidence of "abnormal" behaviors. Furthermore, the most frequent of these behaviors were typical of the patterns described for social isolates, including self-clutching, self-biting, and catatonic limb contractions. The well-fed partial isolate monkeys exhibited some of these behaviors but significantly fewer responses than the malnourished animals reared under identical living conditions.

Table 15.2. Frequency of abnormal behaviors in 70 tests of social behavior

	Group 6	Group 7	Group 8	Group 9
	Low-protein partial isolates	High-protein socially enriched	High-protein partial isolates	Low-protein socially enriched
Self-mouthing	13	0	25	61
Self-clutching	133	1	48	1
Self-biting	394	0	29	3
Inappropriate sex posture	5	1	65	14
Eye poking	12	7	1	11
Catatonic limb	81	0	24	3
Oral homosexuality	0	0	22	418
Masturbation	33	0	21	0

The low-protein (ENR) group also engaged in a high frequency of "abnormal" behaviors but more typically those found in immature monkeys (for example, self-mouthing and oral-genital stimulation). These behaviors have been reported in laboratory-reared animals but usually disappear by the end of the first year in monkeys reared together. The incidence of "abnormal" behavior in the high-protein (ENR) group was almost nonexistent; and comparisons with the low-protein (ENR) monkeys strongly suggest that malnutrition delays or precludes the departure of these immature behaviors with social experience during development.

It might be assumed that the social situation for the malnourished monkeys produces excessive emotionality and physiological arousal. The low-protein (ISO) animals, by this hypothesis, were expected to show heightened stress responses in the social playroom in anticipation or following the adverse nature of peer-peer contact. The increased incidence of abnormal behaviors in the low-protein (ISO) group were also thought to be related to heightened emotionality in these animals. Erwin, Mitchell, and Maple[5] studied self-biting in monkeys that lived primarily in partial isolation but were occasionally paired with another animal. They found that when self-biting occurred it was almost exclusively in association with threats directed toward other animals present, or toward observers. The authors described these occasions as "uncompletable events" implying that self-biting results from frustration.

Gluck and Sackett[9] produced self-biting in partial isolate monkeys by introducing an extinction schedule in a lever-pressing situation. The rate of self-biting decreased with continued extinction trials. One possible interpretation is that self-biting somehow relieves or reduces the stress produced by uncompletable or frustrating events.

The high- and low-protein monkeys were fitted with FM radio transmitters to measure cardiac responses in free-moving social situations. First, electrocardiograms were made from animals sedated with Ketaset and restrained in a primate chair. Figure 15.1 shows the heart rates of the monkeys reared under different diets and living conditions. Neither of the main effects, diet or rearing conditions, were statistically significant under the sedated condition, but the high-protein monkeys had significantly lower heart rates when physically restrained. The cardiac response when the

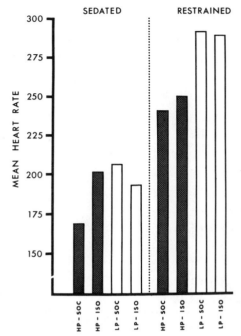

Figure 15.1. Average heart rates (beats per minute) during sedation and restraint

animals were placed in the social playroom alone or with other members of their respective groups are shown in Figure 15.2. Again, statistical significance was obtained only for diet effects, with the high-protein monkeys showing lower overall heart rates. These well-fed controls reared together showed the lowest heart rates of any group, particularly when they were in the presence of cagemates. The high-protein (ENR) monkeys showed significantly lower overall heart rates, despite the fact they more actively engaged in physical exercise (climbing, play, moving about the room), than any of the other groups.

The most interesting results were obtained during observations of self-biting in the low-protein (ISO) group. In all cases (N = 4), the average heart rate increased (80 beats per minute) within four seconds *after* the onset of the "abnormal" behavior. This finding is consistent with the interpretation that self-biting is related to frustration and emotional arousal. However, it does not support the contention that self-biting leads to arousal reduction.

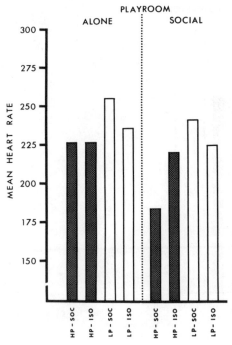

Figure 15.2. Average heart rates in playroom while alone or in a group

In addition to the social playroom observations, learning experiments were conducted on the group-reared and partial isolate monkeys.

It was proposed earlier that the inferior performance of protein-malnourished monkeys on tasks involving stimulus-response discontinuity might reflect a disruption of attentional mechanisms. In the previous studies reported, the critical cues for locating the rewards were present in the stimulus situation, but the malnourished animals failed to locate them readily. A new task, spatial delayed alternation, provided another method for separating the discriminative cues from the response locus. This time the cue to alternate was located internal to the animal.[6] The monkeys were first presented identical grey blocks with food rewards located under both. The animal responded by displacing one of the blocks to obtain the food. On the next trial, food was located under the block that was not selected on the first trial. If the animal failed to alternate to obtain the reinforcer, the trial was rerun until he was successful. When the monkey located the reward, it was moved under the opposite grey block on the subsequent trial. In other words, the adoption of a simple "shift" strategy was all that was required for successful performance of this task. The critical cue was the location of the animal's last response. If the animal perseverated on a single response locus, or failed to attend to the position of his last response, his performance suffered. A time delay ranging between 10 and 60 seconds between trials was instituted to increase the attentional demands placed upon the subject.

No differences were found between malnourished monkeys and controls on the simple delayed response test conducted previously.[34] The critical cue, however, in delayed response is provided directly by the experimenters, and poorer performance on this task is usually interpreted to be the result of deficiencies in short-term memory. Delayed alternation, as suggested, involves more than an effective memory of the correct response over the delay intervals.

The performance comparison of high- and low-protein groups on delayed alternation problems are presented in Figure 15.3 The well-fed controls were originally inferior to the malnourished monkeys but within 15 days surpassed the performance of the low-protein subjects. The terminal levels of successful alternation for the high-protein groups were significantly greater than the levels for the low-protein groups.

The main environmental effects were also found to be significant. Figure 15.4, however, indicates that the performance of the group-reared monkeys was inferior to the performance of the partial isolates. The best performances on delayed alternation were obtained by the high-protein (ISO) animals and the poorest by the low-protein (ENR) monkeys. The correction procedure of the experimental design allowed the subjects to make more than one error on a given problem. An analysis of perseverative errors revealed that the group-reared monkeys made significantly more of these response errors than the partial isolates.

We observed that the group-reared animals appeared agitated in the WGTA and were reluctant to enter the transport cages. One explanation for the poorer performance of these animals is that separation from cage mates for testing was aversive. The individually caged partial isolates were less disrupted when they were transferred to the test cage than the socially reared monkeys

David Strobel

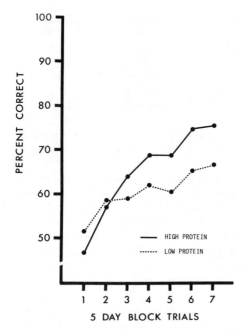

Figure 15.3. Performance on delayed alternation across 5-day block trials (diet conditions)

who were displaced to a completely different environment from the one they were adapted to.

A second learning task presented to these groups involved a simplified version of the reversal problem previously found to differentiate low-protein (DSE) monkeys from high-protein (DSE) monkeys.[34] The modified reversal test was designed by Elias and co-workers at Harvard. Two wooden blocks painted half red and grey or half green and grey were presented to the monkeys in the WGTA, with the colored portions facing the animals. Responses to one specified color were consistently reinforced until the animals reached a criterion of 21 out of 30 correct responses in a row. The previously nonreinforced color block was then rewarded until the monkeys again reached the previous criterion. The reversal problems were made more difficult by turning the grey portion of the stimulus blocks toward the subjects. Because all of the monkeys consistently touched the forward portion of the blocks when responding, a stimulus response discontinuity was present during reversal trials.

Table 15.3 indicates that the rearing condition of the animal had the greatest influence on the original learning of the red/green discrimination problem. The group-reared (ENR) monkeys took significantly more trials to reach criterion than the individually housed animals (ISO). The dietary manipulation, on the other hand, appeared to affect performance on reversal problems. The protein-malnourished monkeys took significantly longer to learn the reversal.

These results support the previous conclusion that learning performance may be greatly altered by the conditions of the testing environment. If these conditions are significantly different from the daily adapted living conditions, early performance on the test problems may suffer. However, experience with the test situation was insufficient to prevent the malnourished subjects from showing decrements in reversal performance.

To further explore the hypothesis that the correspondence between the test and nontest situations is an important variable influencing the test performance of the monkeys reared under dif-

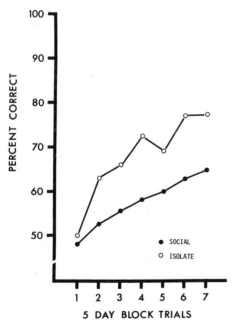

Figure 15.4. Performance on delayed alternation across 5-day block trials (rearing conditions)

Table 15.3. Comparison of average trials to criterion between social rearing and
dietary groups

	Original learning	Reversal
ENR	169	225
ISO	102	218
High protein	139	195
Low protein	132	248

ferent living conditions, a new test apparatus was designed. The
device, Home Cage Test Apparatus (HCTA) was essentially a port-
able WGTA that attached to the living cages of the monkeys. Glass
partitions divided the group living cages so that individual members could be tested separately. The HCTA, thus far, has been used
to test group-reared anemic monkeys on a delayed matching-to-
sample task. Their performance in a WGTA and HCTA were compared. The anemic monkeys were found significantly inferior to
dietary controls when tested in the WGTA, but the differences
disappeared when the same tests were conducted in the home
cages.

Finally, the impact of partial social isolation and protein malnutrition on preference for viewing complex social stimuli was
measured. The monkeys were individually placed in one side of a
double-width chamber. An opaque partition dividing the chamber
contained a hole in the center. Stimuli were projected onto a
screen at the back of the unoccupied half of the chamber so that
the monkeys were required to put their heads through the partition to view the slide. The stimulus objects were 30 black and
white, or colored slides, containing pictures of monkeys or visual
patterns.

The results indicated that the partial isolates viewed all types of
slides with less frequency and duration than group-reared animals. In addition, a significant Diet X Slide Type interaction was
detected. Pictures of monkeys engaged in passive postures or
simple patterns were preferred by low-protein animals over slides
of monkeys exhibiting fear reactions, aggressive postures, and
complex visual patterns.

In sum, malnutrition combined with restricted social rearing
appeared to reduce significantly the visual investigative interests

of monkeys and preferences during slide exploration. In view of the fact that it has often been difficult to find behavioral measures that reveal dramatic differences between diet groups, these results were significant.

Second-generation Protein-malnourished Monkeys

The logical extension of our research to examine the behavioral effects of postnatal malnutrition was to evaluate progressively earlier forms of nutritional insult. Comparisons of prenatal and postnatal malnutrition are critical in view of current discrepancies involving the influence of severity, time of onset, and duration of the nutritional deficiency on learning capacities. The primary factor, however, that advanced our participation in research involving prenatal forms of malnutrition was the successful ability of preadolescent monkeys to adapt to the conditions of severe protein deficiency and to recover relatively unscathed. It was truly a remarkable demonstration of the durability and adaptability of a primate species and suggested the possibility that malnutrition could be studied in early ontogenetic forms.

Before discussing these experiments, however, let us look at preliminary results obtained from low-protein (DSE) monkeys that were rehabilitated after 1,290 days on the protein-deficient diets. These studies ostensibly found the rhesus monkey capable of recovering, both physically and behaviorally, following realimentation. Performance by previously malnourished monkeys on attention tasks (including discrimination reversal problems and pattern string tests) was indistinguishable from controls. Monkeys that had been malnourished continued to show hyperaggression and disrupted social behavior for as long as a year after dietary rehabilitation. Conclusive data from social observations, however, was lacking because of unavoidable disruptions in the testing program. Currently the low-protein (ISO) and low-protein (ENR) groups, described above, are undergoing dietary rehabilitation after 1,500 days on the protein diets. It is hoped that more precise information with respect to the long-term effects of protein malnutrition will be provided in the near future.

Three females from the low-protein (DSE) group were allowed to breed with experienced males following rehabilitation. Approximately 120 days from conception these pregnant females were again placed on the low-protein diets. Two additional pregnant females were also placed on the low-protein diet at the same time in pregnancy. The latter two animals had not experienced protein deficiency prior to this time. A control group of four pregnant females previously reared on standard laboratory chow (15 percent protein) was provided the purified high-protein diet at 120 days of pregnancy.

One of the previously malnourished females had an unsuccessful breech delivery 28 days after the onset of the low-protein diet. The remaining females went full term. The malnourished infants were found to have 96.1 percent the body weight of the controls at birth but only 56.4 percent the weight of well-fed infants at 100 days of age.

Each group of mothers and infants was housed together in a community cage connected by tunnels to a third, empty, but centrally located, cage. Entrance to the tunnels was blocked by a partition containing an orifice sufficiently large for the passage of infants but not the mothers. By 100 days of age, 75 percent of the high-protein monkeys moved freely between the housing cages. None of the malnourished monkeys entered the tunnels at this age.

Mother/infant interactions were observed through a one-way viewing screen when the infants were 100 to 200 days of age. The malnourished infants spent 57 percent of their time attached to their mothers, and controls were observed in contact with their mothers 60.5 percent of the time. While these differences were not found to be statistically significant, qualitative differences in the releasing patterns were observed between the groups. Activities away from the mothers in the high-protein groups were initiated almost exclusively by the infants, whereas the previously malnourished mothers removed their infants from the breast, forcibly rejecting them. One of the doubly deprived mothers was repeatedly observed to reject the infant at the breast, to beat it by rolling and pressing it into the cage floor, and to ignore its distress calls. None of the mothers that were malnourished for the first time at pregnancy demonstrated these abnormal maternal behaviors.

When the infant monkeys were 200 days of age, the mothers were removed from the group cages. Subsequently, the young-animal groups were allowed daily access to the central cage area where chains were suspended from mechanical counters. Chain pulling was measured under three conditions: chains alone, chains with novel objects attached, chains with familiar objects

Behavior and Malnutrition in Nonhuman Primates

attached. Table 15.4 shows the average chain pulls per session for the two groups. A chi square analysis indicated that the high-protein monkeys were significantly more active at chain pulling than the malnourished monkeys ($X^2 = 107.1$, $p < .000001$). The attachment of novel objects to the chains significantly increased chain pulling in both groups, although the dietary controls responded at a frequency more than three times that measured for the malnourished monkeys. On the other hand, familiar objects received little attention by the high-protein subjects, and differences between groups were not statistically significant under this condition.

Another form of manipulative curiosity was measured in the central test cage. Each group was allowed access to a 12-unit puzzle board attached to the wall of the central cage. Puzzle solutions were measured as the number of pin, hook, and hasp combinations manipulated within the 30-minute session. Photocells and counters at the tunnel entrances to the central cage measured the movements to and from the test area. The entrance tunnel to the home cage of the nonparticipating group was blocked with either an opaque partition or a wire mesh screen. Puzzle tests were conducted either with food reinforcement available after successful solution or without appetitive rewards.

The high-protein monkeys were found significantly more active in their movements in and out of the puzzle test cage ($X^2 = 23.02$, $p < .0005$). In addition, the malnourished animals avoided the central test chamber when the entrance to the control group's home cage was blocked only by a screen. The control monkeys were visible through the entrance tunnels under this condition. The high-protein animals appeared more interested in solving the puzzles (not statistically significant) and were more efficient in solving the puzzles than the low-protein monkeys ($X^2 = 262.41$, $p < .00001$). In other words, they solved more puzzles per contact

Table 15.4. Average chain pulls in the central cage for high- and low-protein monkeys

	Chains alone	Chains, familiar objects	Chains, novel objects
Low protein	7.7	47.7	54.0
High protein	79.0	57.3	184.0

211

with the metal surfaces of the puzzles than the malnourished subjects. The introduction of food rewards had little effect on the
puzzle-solving behavior of either group.

Currently the social behavior of these animals is being observed
in the playroom, using categories of behavior modified from a
system developed by Chamove.[2] Selected tasks will be provided
in the near future to test the second-generation malnourished
animals for possible deficiencies in learning performance.

Discussion

Our research program, originally designed to test the short-term
effects of severe, acute, protein malnutrition, was modified to examine long-term protein restrictions from weaning to puberty.
The meaning of "severe" may be described in terms of the degree
of restricted protein content in the diet or by reference to the
ability of the organism to adjust to the dietary restriction. In the
current research, despite the long-term deprivation conditions
and marked growth retardation, only relatively mild behavioral
deficits were produced. The monkeys survived a diet that would
be considered severe by virtue of the protein content but mild-
to-moderate with respect to behavioral consequences. The long-
term good health of the animals reflected the ability of disease-
free monkeys to adapt readily to the conditions of protein malnutrition.

The monkey diets contained 2 to 3.5 percent protein by weight,
which is considerably less than the 7 to 10 percent protein usually
found in diets that effectively produced severe malnutrition in
rats. It would appear that primates, including humans, can thrive
quite nicely on diets containing only 10 percent protein. These
results suggest that serious consideration must be given to the
possibility that different organisms vary in their ability to adjust
physiologically and behaviorally to dietary restriction. It is not
unreasonable to assume that organisms of different phylogenetic
backgrounds evolved with different capacities for adjustment to
dietary imbalance. In sum, our results question the application of
animal models to evaluate the human condition without consideration of phyletic differences in tolerance for low levels of protein intake.

The repeated failures to find deficits in standard tests of discrimination learning, cognitive learning sets, short-term memory,
and reversal learning by protein-malnourished monkeys were ini-

tially puzzling. One possibility is that the postnatal initiation of the protein deficiency was sufficiently past critical periods of brain growth to suggest the sparing of intellectual impairment produced by structural damage. Furthermore, it might be argued that the increased interest by the protein-restricted monkeys for food rewards somehow compensated for performance deficits produced by intellectual impairment. This isn't a particularly persuasive argument in view of data that showed sufficient learning performance without use of food rewards. Further studies revealed that performance in certain classes of learning could be disrupted by malnutrition. Specifically, when the task placed increased demands upon attentional processes, the protein-malnourished animals showed concomitant deficiencies in performance. These effects were found to be transitory and reversible with protein supplementation. The results are consistent with the view that the diets produced a condition equivalent to cerebral dysfunction rather than more permanent structural alterations.

It is popular to interpret performance differences between experimental and control subjects in descriptive terms that imply loss of competency. However, if performance is affected by adaptive processes, the performance of malnourished monkeys was not necessarily "inferior" or "poorer" than controls, but just different. Low-protein animals may be "marching to the beat of a different drummer," with the implication that their subsequent behavior has adaptive value that allows the organism to survive. For example, exploring or manipulating objects that do not lead to food wastes precious energy. Conversely, by decreasing growth rates the animal conserves energy and avoids loss of limited material necessary for survival. Description of the behavioral changes that occurred during malnutrition solely in terms of failure and losses ignores the active processes of adjustment and adaptation that likely accompanied dietary restriction.

Unfortunately, it is not clear how changes in behavior that accompany adaptive processes can be distinguished from those that reflect *failures* of adaptation without teleological reference. Simply, if the behavior helped the animal survive, it was by definition adaptive.

Although the low-protein monkeys were food oriented, they showed more rapid extinction than controls after food was removed. They appeared to be discriminating animals and sensitive to changing reward contingencies. Such behavior has obvious adaptive value. Similarly, the malnourished animals showed evidence of a specific hunger for protein, even when the diets were disguised by flavoring and the source of protein was altered. Furthermore, the dominance of food-seeking or food-oriented behaviors may have precluded the normal development of non-food-oriented activities. By this hypothesis, the patterns of social interaction of malnourished animals would be expected to differ from controls. For example, if the low-protein animals avoided social contact because of a preoccupation with food, it is not unreasonable that they should develop into animals that behaved like monkeys restricted in their social experience. Of course, if the interaction between diet and environmental conditions produced functional isolates, it might be expected that these animals would show the behavioral symptoms of a social isolate. Many of our protein-malnourished animals were strikingly similar in description to animals reared in partial isolation.[19] These similarities included maintenance of infantile responses, aversion to novel stimuli, idiosyncratic or bizarre movement, self-clutching, self-biting, and unstable dominance relationships.

On the other hand, the similarities between the behaviors produced by malnutrition and environmental restrictions may have been coincidental. Fuller,[7] for example, proposed that abnormal social behaviors found in isolated puppies were produced by their inability to attend and respond appropriately to social stimuli. Similarly, Miller and co-workers[18] demonstrated that isolate monkeys did not attend to or were incapable of utilizing the communicative expression of other monkeys. In other words, the malnourished monkeys and social isolates may have in common the disruption of attentional mechanisms.

Other hypotheses have been proposed for mechanisms by which malnutrition may effect the behavioral development of the monkey. Zimmermann et al.,[39] for example, reported that protein-malnourished animals behaved more like well-fed animals their own weight and size than like control animals their own age. The preadolescent low-protein monkeys showed fear by grimacing, crying, clutching, and using other infantile responses to mild threat. In comparison, the high-protein control animals engaged in adultlike reciprocated threat postures and grunting. Malnourished subjects, in addition, showed little sexual activity, while dietary controls engaged in normal grooming, presenting, and mounting. The adequately fed monkeys showed physical evidence of developing secondary sex characteristics including the descent of the testicles in the males, and the appearance of sexual folds with coloration in the females. These characteristics were delayed more than 200 days in the malnourished groups and appeared only following the onset of dietary rehabilitation. Fear and avoidance reactions to novel stimuli and situations are not uncommon in healthy, very young, rhesus monkeys. It is conceivable that emotionality and disrupted attention could reflect the maintenance of infantile behavior patterns in the malnourished animal. More specifically, these results suggest the possible delayed development of information-analyzing systems that allow the organism to assimilate and respond appropriately to new and increasingly more complex informational input.

In summary, the use of animal models has allowed only initial exploration of the complex nutritional variables and environmental factors that may contribute to the behavioral development of the organism. We are currently exploring other specific nutritional deficiencies in the developing monkey, including the effects of prenatal zinc restrictions and iron-deficiency anemia. The preliminary results indicate enough parallels between these deficiencies and protein malnutrition to suggest similar mechanisms of behavioral adjustment. This work, we hope, will lead to more general descriptions of a deprivation syndrome for impoverished organisms.

References

1. Aakre, B., D. A. Strobel, R. R. Zimmermann, and C. R. Geist. Reactions to intrinsic and extrinsic reward in protein malnourished monkeys. *Percept. Motor Skills* 36: 787, 1973.

2. Chamove, A. S. A new primate social behavior category system. *Primates* 15(1): 85, 1974.

3. Deo, M. G., S. K. Sood, and V. Ramalingaswami. Experimental protein deficiency: Pathological features in the rhesus monkey. *Arch. Pathol.* 80: 14, 1965.

4. Dobbing, J. Vulnerable periods in developing brain. In *Applied Neurochemistry*, A. N. Davison and J. Dobbing, eds., Blackwell Scientific Pub., Oxford, 1968, pp. 287–316.

5. Erwin, J., G. Mitchell, and T. Maples. Abnormal behavior in nonisolate-reared rhesus monkeys. *Psychol. Rep.* 33: 515, 1973.

6. French, G. M. Associative problems. In *Behavior of Nonhuman Primates*, I, A. M. Schrier, H. F. Harlow and F. Stollnitz, eds., New York: Academic Press, New York, 1965, pp. 167–209.

7. Fuller, J. L. Experimental deprivation and later behavior. *Science* 158: 1645, 1967.

8. Geist, C. R., R. R. Zimmermann, and D. A. Strobel. Effects of protein-calorie malnutrition on food consumption, weight gain, serum proteins, and activity in the developing rhesus monkey (Macaca mulatta). *Lab. Anim. Sci.* 22: 369, 1972.

9. Gluck, J. P., and G. P. Sackett. Frustration and self-aggression in social isolate rhesus monkeys. *J. Abnorm. Psychol.* 83: 331, 1974.

10. Harlow, H. F., R. O. Dodsworth, and M. K. Harlow. Total social isolation in monkeys. *Proc. Natl. Acad. Sci.* 54: 90, 1965.

11. Harlow, H. F., and M. K. Harlow. The effects of early social deprivation on primates. *Symp. Bel Air, II,* "Desafferentation Experimentales à Cliniques," George and Co., Geneva, Switzerland, 1965, pp. 66–77.

12. Kerr, G. R., and H. A. Waisman. A primate model for the quantitative study of malnutrition. In *Malnutrition, Learning, and Behavior,* N. S. Scrimshaw and J. E. Gordon, eds., M.I.T. Press, Cambridge, Mass., 1968, pp. 240–249.

13. Klein, R. E., O. Gilbert, C. Canosa, and R. DeLeon. Performance of malnourished children in comparison with adequately nourished children. *Annual Meet. Am. Assn. Advan. Sci.,* December, 1969.

14. Levitsky, D., and R. H. Barnes. Malnutrition and animal behavior. In *Nutrition, Development, and Social Behavior,* D. J. Kallen, ed., U.S. DHEW, Publ. No. (NIH) 73-242, Washington, D.C., 1973, pp. 3–14.

15. Locke, K. D., E. A. Locke, G. A. Morgan, and R. R. Zimmermann. Dimensions of social interaction among infant rhesus monkeys. *Psychol. Rep.* 15: 339, 1964.

16. Mason, W. A. The effects of social restriction on the behavior of rhesus monkeys. I. Free social behavior. *J. Comp. Physiol. Psychol.* 53: 582, 1960.

17. Mason, W. A. Motivational factors in psychosocial development. In *Nebraska Symposium on Motivation,* W. J. Arnold and M. M. Page, eds., University of Nebraska Press, Lincoln, Nebr., 1970, pp. 35–68.

18. Miller, R. E., W. F. Caul, and I. A. Mirsky. Communication of affects between feral and socially isolated monkeys. *J. Personal. Soc. Psychol.* 7: 231, 1967.

19. Mitchell, G. D., and D. L. Clark. Long-term effects of social isolation in non-socially adapted rhesus monkeys. *J. Genet. Psychol.* 113: 117, 1968.

20. Ordy, J. M., T. Samorajski, R. R. Zimmermann, and P. M. Rady. Effects of postnatal protein deficiency on weight gain, serum proteins, enzymes, cholesterol, and liver ultrastructure in a subhuman primate (Macaca mulatta). *Am. J. Pathol.* 48: 769, 1966.

21. Platt, B. S. Experimental protein calorie deficiency. In *Calorie Deficiencies and Protein Deficiencies,* R. A. McCance and E. M. Widdowson, eds., Little Brown and Co., Boston, 1968, pp. 237–248.

22. Pond, W. G., R. H. Barnes, R. B. Bradfield, E. Kwong, and L. Krook. Effect of dietary energy intake on protein deficiency symptoms and body composition of baby pigs fed equalized but suboptimal amounts of protein. *J. Nutr.* 85:57, 1965.

23. Ramalingaswami, V., and M. C. Deo. Experimental protein-calorie malnutrition in the rhesus monkey. In *Calorie Deficiencies and Protein Deficiencies*, R. A. McCance and E. M. Widdowson, eds., Little Brown and Co., Boston, 1968, pp. 265–275.

24. Rosenblum, L. A., ed. *Primate Behavior*, I, New York: Academic Press, 1970.

25. Sackett, G. P. Abnormal behavior in laboratory reared rhesus monkeys. In *Abnormal Behavior in Animals*, M. W. Fox, ed., Saunders, New York, 1968, pp. 292–331.

26. Stoffer, G., and R. R. Zimmermann. Development of avoidance learning sets in normal and malnourished monkeys. *Behav. Biol.* 9: 695, 1973.

27. Strobel, D. A., and R. R. Zimmermann. Manipulatory responsiveness in protein malnourished monkeys. *Psychon. Sci.* 24: 19, 1971.

28. Suomi, S. J., H. F. Harlow, and S. D. Kimball. Behavioral effects of prolonged partial social isolation in the rhesus monkey. *Psychol. Rep.* 29: 1171, 1971.

29. Turner, C. H., R. K. Davenport, Jr., and C. Rogers. The effect of early deprivation of the social behavior of adolescent chimpanzees. *Am. J. Psychiat.* 125: 1531, 1969.

30. Wise, L. A. The effects of social experience, protein deprivation, and social coalitions on social dominance of rhesus monkeys. Unpublished Ph.D. Thesis, University of Montana, 1973.

31. Wise, L. A., and R. R. Zimmermann. Shock thresholds of low and high protein reared rhesus monkeys. *Percept. Motor Skills* 36: 674, 1973.

32. Wise, L. A., R. R. Zimmermann, and D. A. Strobel. Dominance measurement of low and high protein reared rhesus macaques. *Behav. Biol.* 8: 77, 1973.

33. Woodruff, C. Nutritional aspects of metabolism, of growth and development. *J. Am. Med. Assn.* 196: 214, 1966.

34. Zimmermann, R. R., C. R. Geist, D. A. Strobel, and T. J. Cleveland. Attention deficiencies in malnourished monkeys. In *Symp. Swedish Nutr. Found.*, XII, Almquist and Wiksell, Uppsala, 1974.

35. Zimmermann, R. R., C. R. Geist, and L. A. Wise. Behavioral development, environmental deprivation, and malnutrition. In *Advances in Psychobiology*, II, G. Newton and A. H. Riesen, eds., John Wiley and Sons, New York, 1974, pp. 133–192.

36. Zimmermann, R. R., P. L. Steere, D. A. Strobel, and H. L. Hom. Abnormal social development of protein-malnourished rhesus monkeys. *J. Abnorm. Psychol.* 80: 125, 1972.

217

37. Zimmermann, R. R., and D. A. Strobel. Effects of protein malnutrition on visual curiosity, manipulation, and social behavior in the infant rhesus monkey. *Proc. 77th Annual Conv. APA,* 1969, pp. 241–242.

38. Zimmermann, R. R., D. A. Strobel, and D. Maguire. Neophobic reactions in protein malnourished infant monkeys. *Proc. 78th Annual Conv. APA,* 1970, pp. 187–188.

39. Zimmermann, R. R., D. A. Strobel, P. L. Steere, and C. R. Geist. Behavior and malnutrition in the rhesus monkey. In *Primate Behavior,* L. Rosenblum, ed., Academic Press, New York, 1975, pp. 241–299.

Malnutrition and Human Behavior: A Backward Glance at an Ongoing Longitudinal Study

Introduction

Writing any kind of history, including the history of an area of scientific investigation, requires the perspective of hindsight. Nevertheless, it is already clear that the seminal period for the study of the effects of malnutrition on human development came during the sixties, when enormous popular and government interest in the possibly detrimental effects of inadequate nutrition resulted in the financing of a number of large-scale projects. In 1965, a group of investigators at the Institute of Nutrition of Central America and Panama (INCAP) in Guatemala began work on a longitudinal study of the relationship between malnutrition and mental development, with preparations that included a survey of methods and techniques for assessing nutritional status, the design of the experimental intervention, and development of a battery of psychological tests appropriate for use with the target population. The study itself was begun in 1969, data has been collected regularly for the past seven years, and preliminary results are now available on children who have been followed through 4 years of age. These results, though preliminary, provide us with an increasingly clear picture, based on large samples, of the impact of mild-to-moderate malnutrition on a variety of aspects of human development. Rather than focusing narrowly on our research findings, we shall attempt in this chapter to discuss our findings in terms of some of the hypotheses and assumptions with which we began the investigation.

In the early 1960's it was widely assumed that protein deficiency was most widespread among the preschool child population in the underdeveloped world. Although investigators frequently referred to protein-calorie malnutrition (PCM), protein deficiency received the major focus of attention, and it was in this context that our work was begun. The original experimental design included six villages, combined in pairs, which were assigned treatment as follows: two villages were to receive a high-protein, high-calorie food supplement; two villages were to receive a control supplement (which ideally would have no food value but would control for the social and interactional factors associated with attending a supplementation center); and two villages were to be controls receiving no supplemental intervention whatsoever. All six villages were to receive curative and preventive medical care.

Almost immediately this design was modified as it became apparent that it would be beyond available funding levels to conduct the study in six villages simultaneously. In response to estimates of available funding, it was decided to continue with only four villages, all of which were to receive some form of treatment. Although there was some uneasiness about the lack of a treatment control, we felt generally comfortable with the issue as protein versus not protein. At this point we made a crucial decision, although none of us appreciated its importance until much later. A high-protein high-calorie supplement was developed and tested, and plans were made to provide two villages with a control supplement containing artificial sweetener rather than sugar. Concurrently, however, increasing attention was being directed toward cyclamates as possibly injurious to health, and as a result, the decision was finally made to design the control supplement so that it contained approximately one-third the calories contained in the high-protein high-calorie supplement and no proteins whatsoever. That decision proved to be extremely important, and allowed us to make a major finding that had not been anticipated when the study began.

Closely related to the design of the experimental treatment was the entire issue of nutritional status and the problem of estimating nutritional status in free-living human populations. In the early period of the longitudinal study we assumed that we could accurately estimate nutritional status based on three types of information: ingestion of the food supplement, home dietary ingestion based on periodic surveys, and anthropometric measurements taken at regular intervals on the study population. Accordingly, precise records were kept on supplement ingestion by pregnant women and preschool-age children; and periodic home dietary surveys and anthropometric measurements were included in the study design. Since morbidity was known to affect the anthropometric status of the children, careful measurements of morbidity in pregnant women and preschool children were also included in the design. As we shall see, several of our initial assumptions regarding the estimation of nutritional status were incorrect.

With respect to the general problem of the measurement of the impact of malnutrition on mental development, the study was originally designed to focus on the preschool years. This reflected an assumption, prevalent in the published literature at that time, that protein deficiency during the preschool years was especially damaging. Although some investigators had speculated on the importance of prenatal and early postnatal life, relatively little attention had actually been paid to this period. Accordingly, in the longitudinal study the focus was on measurement of mental development and nutritional adequacy during the preschool years. In the initial design of the study relatively little attention was paid either to the evaluation of intellectual ability during infancy or to estimates of nutritional status during pregnancy and infancy. Early in 1970 the investigators reviewed the experimental design carefully and made some basic changes, focusing the study on pregnancy and early childhood. Precise measurement was made of the nutritional health status of the mother during pregnancy as well as the nutritional status of the child early in postnatal life. Additional measures of cognitive development during the first year of life were also developed. This turned out to be a very important decision.

From the beginning of the study, emphasis was placed on the importance of the social environment of the child on the assumption that measures of mental development, even in relatively homogeneously appearing villages with relatively little social-structural stratification, would be essentially uninterpretable unless the social environment could be carefully described and measured. Early investigators of the relationship between malnutrition and mental development had paid relatively little attention to the social environment and this, in part, probably caused workers in the sixties to focus on the importance of the preschool period as opposed to the period of early infancy. Emphasis on the social

Robert E. Klein

Table 16.1. Sample size, 1969 to November 30, 1974

Variable	Number of children born into sample	Total number of children observed
Children available	671	1083
Tested for physical growth		
At birth	405	405
At 36 months	330*	581*
Tested for mental development		
At birth	157	157
At 6 months	472	472
At 15 months	452	460
At 24 months	453*	480*
At 36 months	329*	565*

*Up to November 30, 1974.

environment turned out to be an extremely important orientation, and the absence of measures to interpret the environment would have greatly limited interpretability of the longitudinal data in the INCAP study.

Results to Date

The study described here is still in progress, and the data presented are necessarily incomplete. The longitudinal cohort born into the study between 1969 and 1973 has been followed since conception, and sufficient data are currently available on children up to 48 months of age to analyze these data with respect to the question of the relationship between malnutrition and mental development. Table 16.1 presents the sample sizes available for the longitudinal study, that is, children born into the sample beginning in 1969 as well as the total number of children ever observed in this study under age 3. This is the sample for which data will be presented, although we also have data on children first observed between ages 4 and 7.

Food Supplementation and Nutritional Status

Presented in Table 16.2 is the nutrient content per cup for the two supplements employed in this design. The high-protein high-calorie food supplement, referred to here as "atole," appears on the left, and the contents of the "fresco," the calorie-only supplement, are presented on the right. There is clear evidence that both food supplements improved the nutritional status of both the mother and the preschool child. Figure 16.1 presents the percentage of low-birth-weight babies (less than 2.5 kg) by two levels of maternal supplement ingestion. The low group in this figure was made up of women whose total supplement ingestion during pregnancy was less than 20,000 calories, and the high group was made up of those mothers whose supplement ingestion was about 20,000 calories. The percentage of low-birth-weight babies was consistently lower in the better supplemented group, both in villages that received the fresco as well as villages that received the atole supplementation. This impact on low birth weight was due principally to caloric ingestion during pregnancy and was not apparently enhanced by the additional protein available in the atole supplement. In the high-calorie supplementation group the mean additional caloric ingestion of the mothers was approximately 35,000 calories or about 125 calories per day across the course of pregnancy. This same finding has been replicated across successive births to the same mother where the mother was well supplemented during one pregnancy and poorly supplemented during the following pregnancy. Thus, the relationship was not associated with factors peculiar to a particular mother. Neither

Table 16.2. Nutrient content of supplements, per cup*

	Atole	Fresco
Total calories (Kcal)	163	59
Protein (g)	11	
Fats (g)	.7	
Carbohydrates (g)	27	15.3
Ascorbic acid (mg)	4.0	4.0
Calcium (g)	.4	
Phosphorus (g)	.3	
Thiamine (mg)	1.1	1.1
Riboflavin (mg)	1.5	1.5
Niacin (mg)	18.5	18.5
Vitamin A (mg)	1.2	1.2
Iron (mg)	5.4	5.0
Fluor (mg)	.2	.2

*Review date: October 11, 1973; figures rounded to the nearest tenth.

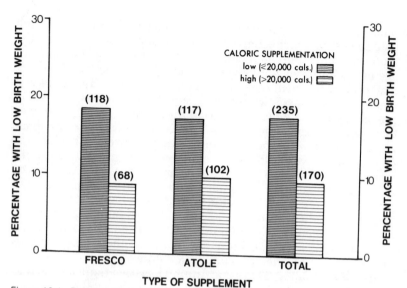

Figure 16.1. Relationship between supplemented calories during pregnancy and proportion of low-birth-weight babies (≤ 2.5 kg)

was the relationship between caloric supplementation and birth weight explained by other maternal variables such as size, home diet, morbidity, obstetrical characteristics, or socioeconomic status.

Figure 16.2 presents data on weight retardation for children born into the longitudinal sample and for whom we have complete data since conception, as was the case with birth weight. The percentage of weight retardation at 36 months of age was strongly associated with calorie supplementation since conception. There was, however, a higher rate of growth retardation in the middle group in the fresco villages than in the atole villages. This difference raises the question of separate effects of proteins and calories on weight gain. This is an important issue, and we are currently exploring it in our data. In spite of this apparent difference, within each of the four villages we found consistent and statistically significant differences in weight gain at 36 months associated with caloric supplementation.

If we were to project the observed differences in this study across the entire seven-year preschool period we would see (Figure 16.3) that approximately half the difference between Guatemalan and North American norms are made up by the food supplement provided to these children. It is our belief that the remaining difference between the projected level of growth in these children and the North American norms is largely due to the high morbidity levels suffered by these children. In contrast with the precision and predictive power of the food supplement for measuring the physical growth of the fetus, infant, and preschool child, the relative amount of information available for estimating the nutritional status of the home diet was a great deal lower. In general we found that the variability in home diets collected in 24-hour recall surveys every three months was simply not powerful enough to improve our estimates of nutritional status based on food supplement ingestion. To improve the precision of the home-diet information would require greatly expanded home-diet survey activity which would ultimately be too costly to justify its use.

Measures of physical growth, in contrast, can be made with great precision and have been taken repeatedly in the present

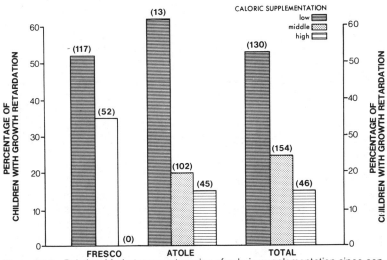

Figure 16.2. Relationship between categories of caloric supplementation since conception and the proportion of children with growth retardation in weight at 36 months of age (n = 330 children born 1969–1973)

225

Robert E. Klein

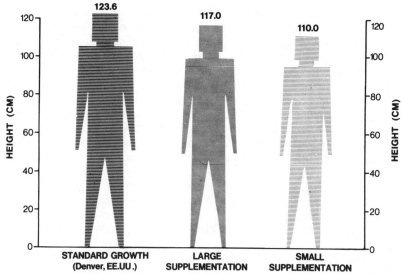

Figure 16.3. Expected heights at 7 years of age of groups given large and small food supplementations

study. However, the percentage of variance in physical growth directly attributable to our measures of nutrient ingestion was relatively small (around 1 to 3 percent). The remaining variance was due at least to other environmental factors—home-diet, morbidity, and to genetic sources. Even to estimate the relative proportions of these two (environment and nutrient ingestion) is not easy (although we are now trying to do so) and to decide that certain small children are undernourished relative to other village children is difficult to prove. Thus, anthropometry for making comparisons within the population now seems much less powerful.

In summary, the supplements employed in the present study were effective in improving the nutritional status, as estimated by birth weight and growth at 3 years of age. The issue of nutritional status and its estimate, originally thought to be possible with considerable precision based on supplement ingestion, home diet, and anthropometric measures has turned out to be somewhat more complicated than originally anticipated. Anthropometric measures served as good indices of the impact of treatment, and treatment was systematically related to these outcome measures.

226

However, home-diet surveys were relatively imprecise for the tasks originally delegated to them. Finally, improvements in nutritional status were associated with calorie ingestion both by the mother and the preschool child, and the additional advantage to protein ingestion at this point seems relatively slight, when discernible at all.

Consistently high levels of ingestion of supplement during the preschool years continued to affect growth across this period in the child's life. Moreover, supplement ingestion was also associated with better psychological test performance. Table 16.3 presents a comparison of mean psychological test performance by level of supplement ingestion as well as the results of analyses of variance by levels of supplement ingestion. The analysis of variance is based on a weighted measure of supplement adequacy in which the number of semesters during which a child or his pregnant or lactating mother was adequately supplemented is summed across the period up to the time of testing. The analysis is for three levels of adequacy. A related correlation analysis based on the total amount of supplement ingestion up to the time of testing also appears in this table. The first variable which appears in the table is from the Brazelton Neonatal Assessment Scale which includes positive signs of vigor, visual following, social interest in examiner, and motor maturity. It will be noted that no relationship is apparent between maternal supplementation during pregnancy and performance on this scale. In other analyses we found relationships both between gestational supplementation and birth weight, as noted earlier, and between birth weight and various measures of the Brazelton Scale.[1] At present both Brazelton and the investigators at INCAP are attempting to construct more adequate summary variables; and research on the relationship between maternal supplementation and neonatal characteristics continues.

The results for the Composite Infant Scale, a collection of items from a variety of standard infant scales, are more clear. By 15 months of age significant relationships between supplement ingestion and performance were apparent, and they were consistent thereafter through 24 months of age. This is the case both for the mental as well as the motor subscales of this test. Item analyses of the individual scales suggest that the impact of supplement ingestion on performance was closely associated with the more motoric and manipulative items both within the mental and motor scales.

Table 16.3. Effect of food supplement ingestion on the Association of Psychological Test Performance up to 36 months of age with supplement ingestion

Psychological test score		S.D. (pooled)	Level of supplement ingestion*			F	Correlation with total ingestion	N†
			Low	Middle	High			
Brazelton Neonatal Assessment								
BG1	$\bar{X}$	13.5	38.83	36.00	39.05	.66	−.042	(157)
	N		42	32	83			
Composite infant scale								
6 months								
Mental	$\bar{X}$	13.8	73.8	76.3	77.8	2.87‡	.030	(472)
	N		150	221	101			
Motor	$\bar{X}$	14.8	70.0	70.6	72.7	1.13	−.017	(472)
	N		150	221	101			
15 months								
Mental	$\bar{X}$	12.5	62.9	67.8	72.3	4.65§	.130§	(460)
	N		140	243	77			
Motor	$\bar{X}$	15.0	73.8	77.2	82.6	6.25§	.134§	(460)
	N		140	248	77			
24 months								
Mental	$\bar{X}$	12.3	61.6	65.5	68.1	8.45§	.161	(480)
	N		206	192	82			
Motor	$\bar{X}$	18.5	67.5	74.4	78.9	11.61§	.221§	(480)
	N		206	192	82			
36 months								
Cognitive composite scale	$\bar{X}$	280.3	−5.28	48.97	54.20	2.75	.060	(565)
	N		278	237	50			
Embedded figures test, sum	$\bar{X}$	3.4	9.43	10.03	9.70	1.91	.069‡	(552)
	N		270	232	50			

Psychological test score		S.D. (pooled)	Level of supplement ingestion*			F	Correlation with total ingestion	N†
			Low	Middle	High			
Embedded figures test, time	X̄ N	11.4	31.5 270	30.1 232	28.9 50	1.58	−.079‡	(552)
Embedded figures test, adaptability	X̄ N	24.0	9.42 270	12.71 232	72.40 50	1.48	.023	(552)
Digit memory	X̄ N	8.3	10.11 224	10.87 232	12.92 50	2.22	.073	(465)
Memory for sentences	X̄ N	12.8	12.06 228	14.22 197	14.60 44	1.85	.076	(486)
Reversal discrimination learning, sum	X̄ N	20.5	23.18 228	23.83 210	20.93 48	.38	−.061	(497)
Reversal discrimination learning, time	X̄ N	11.0	23.4 232	20.7 220	18.3 45	5.13§	−.176§	(497)
Naming	X̄ N	4.3	6.44 262	7.44 220	8.06 45	5.07§	.117§	(539)
Recognition	X̄ N	5.6	19.40 262	20.62 227	20.70 50	2.83‡	.060	(539)
Verbal inferences	X̄ N	1.2	1.25 120	1.52 106	2.08 12	3.28‡	.157§	(238)
Line velocity	X̄ N	45.0	105.9 250	93.4 220	94.4 50	4.84§	−.121§	(520)
Rompecabezas	X̄ N	5.4	5.98 203	5.86 223	6.46 50	.25	.0002	(476)

*See text for definition.
†Sample complete through November 30, 1974.
‡p < .05.
§p < .01.

Robert E. Klein

This is in contrast to the more linguistic or cognitive items in these scales.

At 36 months of age, categories of supplement ingestion were significantly associated with reversal discrimination learning time, vocabulary naming, verbal inferences, and draw-a-line-slowly. In addition, recognition vocabulary showed a marginally significant (p < .10) effect.

Table 16.4 presents the means, f ratios, and correlational values

Table 16.4. Means and standard deviations of psychological test scores by supplementation ingestion category, and anova for nutritional effects

Test	Nutritional status category			F	S.D. (pooled)	Sig. level
	0 $\overline{X}$	1 $\overline{X}$	2 $\overline{X}$			
48 Months						
EFT, sum	4.63 (205)	4.83 (236)	5.55 (31)	1.74	2.60	NS
EFT, time	2.90 (205)	2.69 (236)	2.85 (31)	1.54	1.24	NS
EFT, adaptability	.022 (205)	.054 (236)	.024 (31)	2.02	.175	NS
Digit span	21.05 (200)	21.43 (233)	19.24 (29)	.409	12.37	NS
Sentence span	30.07 (204)	34.10 (231)	36.07 (28)	2.62	20.37	<.100
RDL, sum	33.48 (209)	37.93 (240)	40.97 (31)	3.69	20.15	<.050
RDL, time	1.69 (209)	1.55 (240)	1.58 (31)	2.66	.64	<.100
Vocabulary naming	11.70 (212)	13.89 (238)	14.10 (30)	11.18	5.19	<.005
Vocabulary recognition	25.59 (212)	27.30 (238)	26.63 (30)	5.83	5.35	<.005
Verbal inferences	2.76 (155)	3.05 (191)	3.00 (23)	1.50	1.54	NS
Draw-a-line slowly (cm/sec)	7.30 (203)	5.97 (229)	4.44 (31)	9.65	4.18	NS
Rompecabezas	9.01 (184)	9.06 (236)	8.00 (31)	.359	6.62	NS
Cognitive composite scale	-17.53 (215)	56.52 (241)	67.87 (31)	4.08	291.50	<.025

for supplement ingestion and psychological test performance at 48 months of age. At 48 months of age more tests showed significant associations with categories of supplement ingestion. These included vocabulary naming and vocabulary recognition, number of correct responses on a reversal discrimination learning task, draw-a-line-slowly, and the overall cognitive composite score which is a summary measure of several of the cognitive tests in the battery. In addition, sentence memory and reversal discrimination learning response time were marginally significant at the $p < .10$ level.

The interactions of test performance during infancy and during the preschool ages of 36 and 48 months were explored for a number of variables. The sex of the child was not systematically related to performance differences at any age nor were the effects of attendance to supplementation centers nor varying levels of morbidity in the children.

Thus, in summary, we found systematic relationships from 15 months onward between supplement ingestion and psychological test performance up to the age of 48 months. These results were unrelated to any of the conceivable intervening variables that we were measuring and seemed to be directly associated with calorie ingestion, since the same effects were seen across both atole and fresco villages and were related to the number of calories ingested, rather than proteins as was originally thought to be the case.

Having found that caloric supplement ingestion was associated with better fetal, infant, and preschool physical growth as well as psychological test performance during this period of time, we next examined the question of the relative importance of the timing of food supplement ingestion on psychological test performance. Hypotheses have been advanced for a variety of mechanisms by which improved nutrition might have an impact on psychological test performance,[2] and the present data provide a unique opportunity to put some of these mechanisms to empirical test. Table 16.5 presents correlations as well as partial correlations for the mental subscale and the composite infant scale at 6, 15, and 24 months and for the cognitive composite measure and the verbal inference test at 36 months of age separately for boys and girls. Column 1 presents the simple correlations between the total supplement ingested by the mother during pregnancy and the child's test performances at the ages indicated; column 2 pre-

Table 16.5. Effect of timing of food supplement ingestion on the Association of Psychological Test Performance

Test	I With supplement ingested during pregnancy		II With total supplement ingested to time of testing		III With total supplement ingested to time of testing (II), controlling for supplement ingested during pregnancy (I)		IV With supplement ingested during pregnancy (I), controlling for postnatal supplement ingested to time of testing (II)	
	Boys	Girls	Boys	Girls	Boys	Girls	Boys	Girls
Composite infant scale = mental subscale (at 6 mos.)	.11	.13*	.04	.01	-.07	-.18†	.13*	.15*
Composite infant scale = mental subscale (at 15 mos.)	.09	.24†	.14*	.12*	.11	-.07	.01	.22*
Composite infant scale = mental subscale (at 24 mos.)	.20†	.15*	.19†	.13*	.11	.04	.12*	.09
Cognitive composite scale (at 36 mos.)	.09	.11	.04	.10	.00	.04	.12*	.05
Verbal inference (at 36 mos.)	.36†	.25†	.20†	.12*	.04	-.03	.33†	.23†

*p < .05.
†p < .01.

sents the correlations between the total cumulative supplement ingested by the child and the mother up to the time of psychological testing; column 3 presents the partial correlations of cumulative supplementation with test performances, when maternal supplementation during pregnancy was controlled for; and column 4 shows the correlation of supplement ingested during pregnancy with the child's test performances controlling for postnatal supplementation. It will be noted that the correlations between maternal supplementation ingestion during pregnancy and later test performances are significant, and that when gestational supplementation is partialled out of the correlation between total cumulative supplementation and test scores virtually no relationship remains. In contrast, the association between prenatal maternal supplementation and subsequent test performance is not changed by controlling for later supplementation. This pattern is generally consistent across the ages represented in this table, and is generally consistent for both boys and girls. Our interpretation of these data is that gestation represents a crucial period insofar as effects of supplementation on subsequent psychological test performances up to 36 months is concerned, and that supplement ingestion following birth has relatively little impact on the variables we have measured thus far.

We examined this same pattern by comparing siblings whose mothers ingested different amounts of supplement across successive pregnancies. This analysis has the obvious advantage of controlling for potentially confounding variables which are constant within families. The results are generally similar and support our interpretation that maternal caloric supplementation during pregnancy affects psychological test performances of children, up to 36 months of age.

It is important to keep in mind that the microenvironment of the child and its relationship to his intellectual development is much more varied and complicated than his nutritional or health status. From the earliest period in the study described here, there has been a concern about the impact of the child's microsocial environment and a firm conviction that, unless important dimensions of this environment were accurately measured, the relationship between malnutrition and mental development could not be adequately understood. Early in the study, social structural variables were measured at the family level, and scales were built that combined ratings of each family's house (number of rooms, type of construction), parents' clothing, and the reported amount of direct teaching of preschool children by parents and older siblings. This socioeconomic status scale, which we shall refer to as the Composite SES Scale, was further standardized within villages, to control for intervillage differences in housing style, due to climate and other factors, and was then averaged across three surveys spanning the last five years. The results presented here are based on this overall composite scale which characterizes family characteristics of the children in the sample.

A variety of analyses have been carried out in order to better understand psychological test performances in the context of social structural characteristics of the families of the study children. These analyses are still in progress, but the results to date can be summarized. First, we found no systematic differences across the supplementation groups as a function of the social characteristics of the family. This is to say that supplement ingestion was not related to scores on the family SES scale. In examining the relationships between psychological test performance during infancy and the early preschool years and family sociocultural status, we found that there was relatively little impact on performance before 36 months of age. However, at this time several tests showed significant relationships between supplementation ingestion and performance, but only in the low SES groups. These patterns were fairly complicated and differed somewhat by the sex of the child. Among low SES boys, embedded figures sum correct, adaptability, reversal discrimination learning, response time, and vocabulary recognition were all related to supplement ingestion. Performances for these variables were not related to supplement ingestion among high SES boys. Among low SES girls, but not among high SES girls, embedded figures, adaptability, and reversal discrimination learning time were associated with supplement ingestion.

This interaction between psychological test performance, family social status, and supplement ingestion can be most clearly seen in the context of contingency tables which express performance in terms of relative risk of being in the lowest or highest categories of test performance as a function of nutritional supplementation categories. Table 16.6 presents the results broken down in this fashion for the cognitive composite at 36 months of age. The entire sample is broken down into the lowest and highest pentiles and the middle 60 percent of the sample—which

Table 16.6. Relative risk of falling into extreme 20 percent according to supplementation ingestion and socioeconomic status (SES), derived from cognitive composite made at 36 months

	Number in test performance group				Percentages				Chi-Square		
	Low*	Med.†	High‡	Total	Low	Med.	High	Total	χ	d.f.	P
Total sample											
0	67	162	49	278	24	58	18	100	5.9	4	NS
1	39	145	53	237	16	61	22	99			
2	8	31	11	50	16	62	22	100			
Total	114	338	113	565	22	60	20	102			
Low SES											
0	39	71	13	123	32	58	11	101	10.1	4	<.05
1	22	72	26	120	18	60	22	100			
2	4	16	5	25	16	64	20	100			
Total	65	159	44	268	24	59	16	99			
High SES											
0	26	88	36	150	17	59	24	100	.5	4	NS
1	17	73	26	116	15	63	22	100			
2	4	15	6	25	16	60	24	100			
Total	67	176	68	291	16	60	23	99			

*Lowest pentile.
†Middle 60 percent of scores.
‡Highest pentile.

appear on the left hand side of the table. Percentages for these numbers appear on the right hand side of Table 16.6. Immediately below, the same sample is broken out by levels of SES so that one can examine the relative risk of being in the lowest versus the highest pentile of performers by level of supplementation ingestion separately for low and high SES groups. In the high SES group a poorly supplemented child was about equally likely to fall into the low or high percentiles (17 percent vs. 24 percent). In contrast, among the low SES group, a poorly supplemented child was approximately three times as likely to be in the low as opposed to the high-percent high-pentile group (32 percent vs. 11 percent). This is a vivid example of the general statement that nutritional deprivation and its relationship to mental test performance cannot be understood clearly except in the context of the child's microfamily social environment.

Robert E. Klein

Discussion

In the present paper we have presented some preliminary findings. These data were generated by a research design substantially changed since the study was originally conceived ten years ago. However, in many respects the earlier assumptions which dictated features of the original design have either proven valid or produced unexpectedly valuable data. In general, the results to date reflect important effects of mild-to-moderate malnutrition on mental development. These results also indicate that the nutritional impact can be best understood in combination with measures of the social environment in which the child is being raised. We are extremely fortunate in having designed a powerful experimental treatment, since many of the assumptions about the ability to estimate nutritional status based on measurements of home diet and anthropometry were simply not correct. In spite of this, we were able to document a clear relationship between caloric supplementation during pregnancy and physical growth of the fetus, infant, and preschool child. Similarly, caloric supplementation during pregnancy was significantly related to test performance up to 48 months of age, the oldest age group for which we currently have sample sizes sufficiently large to test this association.

The initial design of the supplement and the crucial decision to include carbohydrates in the fresco rather than cyclamates were responsible for our being able to demonstrate the effect of caloric supplementation. Had cyclamates or some other artificial sweetener been used in the fresco it would have been impossible to separate calories from proteins, and the most likely interpretation would have been that protein was the important factor in physical growth and psychological test performance.

Similarly, the decision in 1970 to strengthen the design in terms of the measures taken during infancy was also crucial in the subsequent interpretation of these data. In 1970 we greatly expanded the number of measures in nutritional status as well as in psychological test performance which were focused on the early period following conception. Had we not greatly expanded the measures of the gestational period we would not have been in the position to identify the importance of gestational caloric supplementation on later psychological test performance.

Finally, our early assumptions about the importance of the so-

236

cial environment of the child in the interpretation of the results were borne out. It is important to note here that the measures used were somewhat gross, and reflected generally the economic conditions of the family and their reported child-rearing practices. In spite of this, these simple measures were powerful aids in interpreting the impact of malnutrition and nutritional supplementation on psychological test performance. It might be expected that sociocultural measures which were theoretically more closely related to psychological test performance, such as the linguistic climate of the home, parental attitudes, and child-rearing practices based on observational measures rather than parents' reports, would additionally enhance the interpretative power of this kind of social-psychological variable. Parenthetically, we have subsequently devoted considerable time and effort to the pursuit of additional and theoretically more functional variables, and we hope to be able to report the results of this effort before too much longer.

References

1. Brazelton, T. Berry. *Neonatal Behavioral Assessment Scale.* J. B. Lippincott, Philadelphia, 1973.
2. Yarbrough, C., R. E. Lasky, J-P. Habicht, and R. E. Klein. Testing for mental development. In *Symp. Swedish Nutr. Found.*, XII, Almquist and Wiksell, Uppsala, 1974, pp. 7–12.

Adolfo Chávez and Celia Martínez 17

Consequences of Insufficient Nutrition on Child Character and Behavior

The Problem in Developing Areas

The proportion of children who grow up undernourished in social environments with limited resources is unknown. Through cross-section surveys in certain areas of the underdeveloped world it has been found that from 25 to 30 percent of the children weigh 25 percent less than the accepted standard for their ages.[1] These figures can be only an estimate, mainly because the groups in which the studies have been made are quite heterogeneous as to age. When the Mexican Nutrition Institute maintained under observation a number of children from birth through 5 years of age, results showed that second- or third-degree malnutrition occurs much more frequently than the surveys indicated. Probably as many as two-thirds of the children studied, at a given moment during their lives, present marked deficiency in weight gain and evident signs of malnutrition.[7]

This high incidence of malnutrition may be explained by the poor practices in child feeding and care that are prevalent in an economically and educationally deprived environment.[6] For the most part, in the poorly developed regions of the world, with the possible exception of certain areas of Africa, it is common practice to feed the child at the breast for an extended period, with but scant and tardy supplementation.[11] Thus the child is limited in his consumption of food from an early age, for it is known that most mothers do not increase their milk production in proportion to the increasing needs of the child.[5]

With a reduction in his protein-calorie supply, the child must

238

use a series of adaptation mechanisms in order to survive, and the principal adaptation seems to be a reduction in growth rate. Thus, for our purposes, the best way to determine the frequency of malnutrition is to measure the growth of the child.[14]

The effect of malnutrition on growth has been known for a long time, but only recently has inquiry been made into its other consequences, which are multiple in nature and affect not only weight and height, but limit also the development of every faculty and potentiality.[10]

Unfortunately, sufficient and adequate studies have not been made among adults that grew up in deprived environments. There are, moreover, many controversies regarding the methodology employed in the few studies that have been made. The type of test used in a poor rural area of Mexico would not be applicable to the urban environment of New York, because the individual experiences in each of these places are necessarily different. It is well known that the behavior of an individual is conditioned not only by his intellectual development and the maturity of his personality, but also by his cultural environment. When differences of opinion arise in this respect, certain social and political aspects come up. It becomes difficult to maintain that individuals coming from a given deprived environment have been unable to develop fully their mental and social capacities because of insufficient nutrition—which is itself a consequence of inequality. The problem should be dealt with from a strictly scientific point of view, putting prejudice aside, in view of its importance to the planning of integral health programs to promote maximum human development.

Of all aspects of human development, perhaps the least known is that relating to the behavioral development of deprived populations. Rather, money, time, and interest are expended today in the study of the behavioral development of several other species of animals, from which, it is hoped, will come useful information for the human species.

There is information available which shows that rural populations of limited resources are apathetic and passive, and have low levels of anxiety and emotional tension. Some people believe this to be good, considering them to be happy in their poverty, whereas others believe that this tranquility and submission are manifestations of a deep-seated social disease.[10] Undoubtedly a person in such circumstances, lacking the opportunity for self expression or introspection and of consciously relating to the environment, and without the possibilities of free choice of his goals in life, of social and self-fulfillment and of attaining emotional maturity, never should be considered a healthy person.

Hypothesis and Experimental Design

The hypothesis for this present study and the basic ideas for its design arose from a previous study made by the authors in the San Jorge Nuchita community—one of the poorest in Mexico—between the years 1965 and 1967. The purpose was to evaluate the possibilities of change in the feeding levels of young children and to measure the effect upon growth in a deprived environment.[2] It was proven that change was possible and that the families could better feed their children despite their limitations. Surprisingly, a change in the nutritional status of the child brought about certain changes in family behavior.[12]

As a consequence of the foregoing, a new study was undertaken. An effort was made to develop an experimental design capable of proving the hypothesis that "an improvement in the nutritional status of a group of children, even without modifying the environment, causes positive change in their physical and mental development and also in their behavior."

The design was based on the measurement of the effect, when introduced into a group of mother-child units, of one variable (better food consumption) upon another variable (development and behavior of the group). The evaluation of the change was obtained by comparison with that of a control group, as similar as possible, without any intentional modification.

In designing the study it was necessary to look for a suitable community, as homogeneous as possible, isolated from external influences, poor, and with the typical feeding patterns of prolonged breast-feeding and late supplementation for the child.

In 1968 the control group of mother-child units was selected. For them, no supplementation was provided, in accordance with the program design. The units conformed to certain standardization criteria, such as follows: the mother had from 1 to 4 children; had a height of from 1.38 m to 1.50 m; was aged 18 to 34 years and healthy; belonged to the peasant social stratum of the community; her child at birth was normal and weighed from 2,500 g to 3,400 g.

When this group was integrated, women possessing characteristics similar to the foregoing were selected for the experimental group. Supplementation was then begun, following approximately the 45th day of pregnancy, with 3 daily rations of powdered milk and sufficient vitamins and minerals. Upon the birth of the child, if he or she possessed the characteristics allowing for the pairing of this mother-child unit with a pair from the control group, supplementation of the mother was continued throughout lactation, and supplementation of the child with the necessary foodstuffs was begun from the moment that this was considered indicated. The core sample that has been analyzed for this report corresponds to the first 3 years of life of 17 pairs, as a loss of 3 pairs resulted in each group.

When the experimental design was planned, a total purity of the system was not expected because this is impossible to obtain among humans. For example, there will always be the effect of contact with the researcher and the particular bias on the part of the investigators to "expect a certain effect," and so on. An effort was made at all times to achieve standardization, and "blind systems" were employed. These objectives were attained within certain limits. For all practical purposes they appear to have been quite adequate.

Although the findings showed a positive improvement in health status as a result of supplementation, reaching normality in certain aspects, the experimental group could not be termed essentially "well nourished," since all factors involved had not been checked. For that matter, the control group could not be referred to as "malnourished," for these children were not, strictly speaking, ill. In fact, those individuals who became clinically malnourished were treated immediately and removed from the study because of the intervention. For this reason, throughout the study, reference is always made either to the "supplemented" or the "nonsupplemented" group, with the nutritional implications that this may reveal, and not to the "well nourished" or "malnourished."

Another very important consideration is that although this study was designed primarily to intervene with the purpose of modifying only one variable, "nutrition," other factors came into play, such as, for example, collaterals in foods. This variable is complex, since food is not only a source of nutrients, but also supplies greatly varying types of stimuli, several of which were detected early in the course of the investigation, were observed longitudinally, and are now presented in this paper.

241

Methodology of the Investigation

In order to make sure that the experimental group had been adequately supplemented, very detailed studies were made regarding food consumption, particularly that of the child.[13] Consequently, it was possible to demonstrate the effect of supplementation upon variables such as growth and health.[7]

The behavior of the child was evaluated through 4 different procedures:

1. Formal tests, of the Gessel type, were applied monthly during the first year of life of the child and quarterly thereafter.

2. Evaluation was made of mother-child interaction by direct observation within the home, employing a system of systematic sampling in time.[3] Every 2 months for the first year and every 4 months thereafter, 17 objective aspects of mother-child interaction were observed. Photographs were taken at intervals of 30 seconds between observations for periods of 150 minutes in the morning and for 150 minutes in the evening. As some areas were considered irregular in their presentation, particularly the physical activity of the child and his interaction with his father, other types of sampling in time were also carried out, taken for periods of 10 minutes on the hour throughout the whole day.

3. A special questionnaire was prepared to obtain the scalographic classification of 31 indicators covering the effect of the environment upon the child. Therein were graded various family situations, at different hours of the day or night, seeking out and qualifying certain behavioral patterns, such as, for example, habits of cleanliness, accident prevention, educative instructions given, stimuli, prizes, concessions made, and so on. All these areas of behavior were evaluated longitudinally, some qualitatively, and others quantitatively.[9]

4. Tests were designed to measure the dependence-independence system of the child in an open-field controlled situation with the following procedure: the child was placed in the centre of a 3 m by 3 m checker board style square, with the mother at one side and toys in front, while the observers, on the sides, took note of the displacement of the child per check marked out on the floor.[8]

Behavior of the Supplemented Experimental Group

The supplemented children exhibited important differences from 24 weeks of age. For example, they slept less during the day, were not resigned to remaining in the cradle, even when rocked, and preferred to stay out of doors (Figure 17.1).

Other aspects, in which observation through sampling in time showed differences, were revealed when supplemented children, after 24 weeks of age, refused to be carried on their mothers' backs or to be rolled up in the "rebozo," and preferred to be free, playing in the yard with their brothers and sisters.

This method of sampling in time also showed that after 72 weeks of age there was a great difference in mother-child proximity. Whereas the supplemented child kept away from the mother, the nonsupplemented stayed close to the mother, and very often was observed being carried either in arms or on the back.

The most notable difference brought out by the method of sampling was that relating to the physical activity of the child. At one year of age, the supplemented child was 3 times as active, and at 2 years of age as much as 6 times as active.[4]

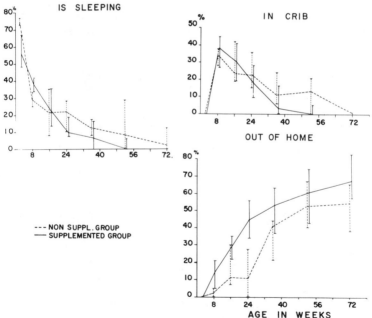

Figure 17.1. Percent of observation in which subjects were observed sleeping, in crib or out of home, as a function of dietary supplementation and age

The scalographic system of analysis, using indicators of the family-child relationship, shows that the supplemented children got more attention from their mothers and from the rest of the family. For example, they were both cleaned and washed more frequently, and they also received more immediate attention when they demanded it (Figure 17.2).

The mother was also more concerned about the child and adopted more protective measures to avoid his getting burnt or bruised, or injured by falling out of the cradle (Figure 17.3). Despite this, there were several accidents recorded among supplemented children, one of them fatal.

From 36 weeks, various attitudes of deference toward the child were apparent. For example, the child was spoken to more frequently and was often praised. The parents were proud of this child, who was rewarded with presents, toys, and clothing. More attention and consideration were bestowed progressively on the supplemented children, and more emotional contact was had

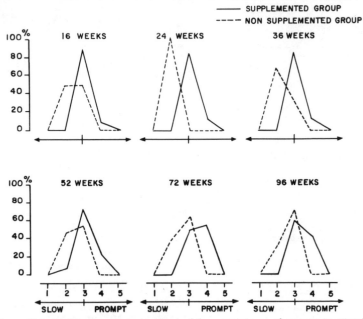

Figure 17.2. Distribution of observations of the promptness of parents to attend to child's demands as a function of age and supplementation

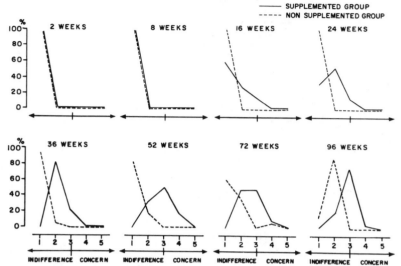

Figure 17.3. Distribution of observations of parental concern of hazards to child as a function of age and supplementation

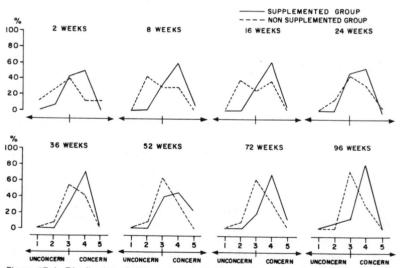

Figure 17.4. Distribution of observations of father's concern toward child as a function of age and supplementation

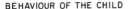

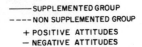

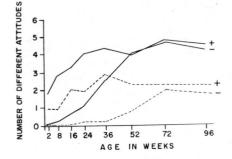

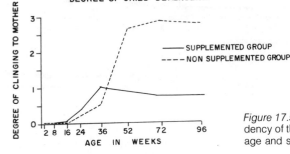

Figure 17.5. Attitude and dependency of the child as a function of age and supplementation

with them. Generally speaking, supplemented children were offered more stimuli. For example, the mothers were already speaking to them, smiling at them, and playing with them at 6 months of age. In the nonsupplemented children this level was attained only when they reached 2 years of age.

In general, in the rural communities of Mexico, fathers are not in the habit of sharing in the care of their children. Thus the finding, that in a large proportion of cases among the supplemented, the fathers did play with their children, proved to be a very outstanding change. After the first year of age, more than half of the fathers began to share in a considerably varied interaction with the children, such as speaking to them, or carrying and

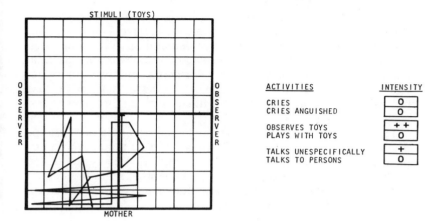

Figure 17.6. Example of test of physical activity of child

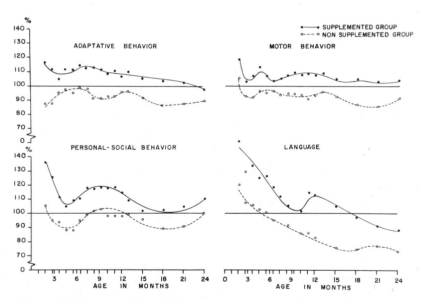

Figure 17.7. Results of Gesell Test Performance as a function of age and supplementation

playing with them (Figure 17.4). Differences in behavior began to appear between the two groups of children. Supplemented children appeared, on the one hand, more expressive, charming, and playful, but on the other were more demanding and headstrong. In time they tended to become more touchy, aggressive, and independent (Figure 17.5). They also became progressively more detached from the mother and tended to associate more with their fathers, brothers, and sisters, and liked to play more in the yard with the animals.

The results of open-field tests were very different in both groups of children. The supplemented appeared to be much more curious, active, and aggressive (Figure 17.6). The nonsupplemented were much more passive, sought out the mother more frequently, and explored the environment less often. They scarcely ever approached the toys and were very insecure when submitted to the field test.

The Gessel tests also showed differences, particularly in the area of speech and social-personal behavior (Figure 17.7). At certain ages there were great differences between the groups; at other ages there was an adjustment, and differences diminished significantly.[9]

Behavior of the Nonsupplemented Control Group

Although in the design of the project the nonsupplemented group was considered the control group, basically it became the target group of the investigation, for it was precisely an evaluation of the behavior patterns of a group like this which was needed to prove the null hypothesis that "the behavior of the deprived child, whoever he may be, is the primary consequence of lack of food." By design, then, nutrition was separated from other components of the poverty complex.

Among the multiple manifestations which might be attributed to the nutrition variable, the most outstanding were insufficient growth and practically no increase over time in the physical activity of the child (Figure 17.8). For an extended period, even up to the age of 3, the child spent much of his time asleep in his cradle in the darkness of his home, very often with his face covered by a netting, or wrapped up and carried on his mother's shoulder. As late as 72 weeks of age, crying continued to be best means of communication with the mother and served to secure that which was most satisfying to him, his mother's breast. This turned out to

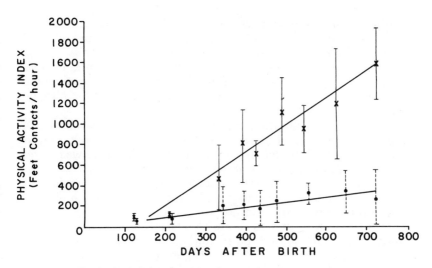

Physical activity (average feet contacts per hour) at different
ages in non supplemented (-•-) and supplemented (-x-) groups.

Figure 17.8. Amount physical activity (feet contacts) in infants as a function of age
and supplementation

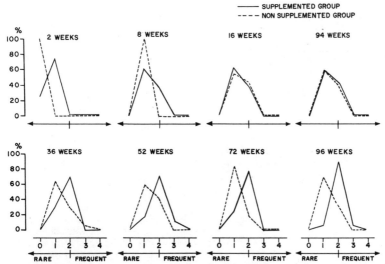

Figure 17.9. Distribution of observations of direct stimuli as a function of age and
supplementation

be the instrument of contact and stimulation and was the highest prize that the mother could give to the child. Every time the child cried, the mother responded by giving it the breast for as long as he wished, and even though he did not get enough milk, he held it, nibbling on it for periods of up to 45 minutes. Every time the child cried he got the breast, and if he asked for nothing else, he got nothing else (Figure 17.9).

The method of sampling in time showed that at 72 weeks of age the nonsupplemented child rarely talked and very rarely played (Figure 17.10). Fifty-five percent of the time the child was quiet, close to his mother, and at times was clutching her skirt.

It became evident that the mother really had concern for the child, but she lacked initiative and did not know how to play an active role. If the child did not ask for food or toys, she did not give them to him. It was found, for example, that she did not impart important stimuli, particularly of the verbal type, or educate the child actively (Figure 17.11), even up to the age of 2.

At 36 weeks, which is when a child begins to be active, the

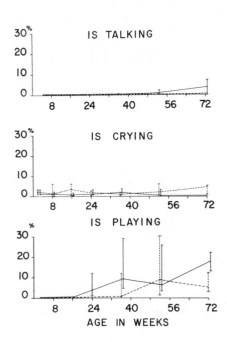

Figure 17.10. Percent of observations that child was observed talking, crying, or playing as a function of age and supplementation (———: supplemented group; ----: nonsupplemented group)

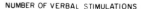

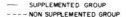

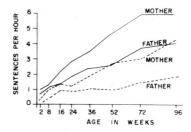

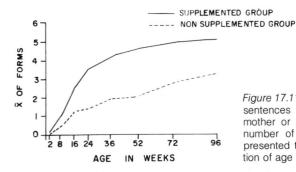

Figure 17.11. Mean number of sentences spoken to child by mother or father and the mean number of forms of stimulation presented to children as a function of age and supplementation

nonsupplemented child tried to clutch the mother and in the open-field tests frequently showed great anxiety and fear when left in the middle of the checkerboard pattern on the floor. He made no effort to see or look for anything. Very often he did not even make a move toward his mother, but just sat in despair demanding that his mother come for him.

In general, the behavior of the nonsupplemented children may be defined as quiet, reserved, and timid. They had great difficulty in making up their minds and, once the decision was made, began any movement very slowly; but at times, when they had managed to calm down, they were able to perform the movement correctly.

Adolfo Chávez and Celia Martínez

Mechanism of the Relation between Nutrition and Behavior

The experimental design allowed for demonstration of the effect of supplementation upon behavior for, although 100 percent purity was not achieved in the design, it may be maintained that the majority of the control systems of interconcurrent variables— that might have been factors for secondary modifications— worked well.

What did stand out, was that supplementation constituted a complex, and was not just calories and proteins. Conspicuously outstanding was the effect upon the child of the knowledge that there were alternatives to the breast, meaning other sources of satisfaction often as gratifying as the breast. Also, the exogenous supplements given to the mother-child system allowed for a different kind of contact between the mother and the child, as well as yet another with the research auxiliaries from the project. Food was not the only variable: the child was almost 30 percent less days ill, larger in size, could get around sooner, and above all had more energy for physical activity. Nevertheless all these must come under the variable "supplementation," for all previously discussed components belong to its very essence.

The design, to a great extent, made it possible to prove the hypothesis that "food modifies behavior." It also confirmed our belief that insufficient nutrition is the principal factor of a deprived environment, affecting the personality, limiting it to a passive, negative, and dependent one. Observations in this study suggest the following chain of events as the central line of the behavioral conditioning system: more food makes for a more active child, who becomes more demanding and interacts more with both mother and family. The family is obliged to respond, and in so doing, creates a new dimension of interaction, at a higher level of stimulation. This makes for better brain functioning in the child and consequently a more mature personality.

This sequence cannot be demonstrated, although it was observed. It is also apparent that many other factors may be involved. In the open-field test a rather striking behavior pattern occurred which may be considered as characteristic and singular of each child and possibly related to origin. From a very early age every child followed a peculiar pattern of action when moving about over the checkerboard square, a pattern which neither time nor nutrition could change. Perhaps this particular behavioral trait belongs to the dominance-security system found in primates.[15]

It cannot be denied that many other such environmental factors, including illness, form a complex which makes discernment difficult. Nevertheless, it was obvious to the investigators that physical activity was what prompted the mother to closer contact with the child. For example, she saw to it, from a very early age, that the child did not fall out of the cradle because of its unusual activity. It was also evident that the physical activity of the child induced the father to give a hand and that his playfulness made his brothers and sisters play the more with him. Some mothers, unaccustomed to such an active and demanding child, sought help from the investigators, recognizing that their homes were inadequate and even dangerous for sheltering such an active child.

It may be said that the active child works upon his environment, provoking more stimuli upon himself and interacting with it. This proves that a child contributes substantially to creating his own environment, even within such a limited one as that studied here.

Many other variables, however, in addition to physical activity, may have an important role in this situation. For example, the fact that the supplemented child was larger modified his interaction with his mother, who eventually found difficulty in carrying him. His more grown-up appearance resulted in his being treated differently by the family, who no longer thought of him as a baby.

Certain practices, such as bathing and changing the baby more frequently, may be related to the fact that his body temperature was higher and he had more abundant perspiration. Preliminary investigations appear to bear this out. It must be remembered that the mother was also supplemented from pregnancy and probably throughout lactation. This may have resulted in better health for her and greater capability for child care.

Nevertheless, neither physical activity nor many of the differences mentioned explain certain aspects of the character of the children. Why were the nonsupplemented children negative, withdrawn, and timid, whereas the supplemented were more playful, charming, demanding, and aggressive? Why did the nonsupplemented child, at 72 weeks of age, revert to a position of fear of facing the environment? It is possible that the differences in the experiences of both groups may have been responsible, on the one hand, for the frustrated and deprived nonsupplemented child

Adolfo Chávez and Celia Martínez

being withdrawn, and, on the other hand, for the satisfied supplemented child seeking out with more aplomb and self-assurance an ever increasing degree of independence.

These aspects, of great interest to workers concerned with the behavioral consequences of human deprivation and its core problem—which we considered to be insufficient nutrition—are the ones on which the research group is presently concentrating.

References

1. Bengoa, J. M. Nutritional significance of mortality statistics. *Proc. Western Hemis. Nutr. Congr.*, III, Futura Pub. Co., Miami, 1971, p. 270.
2. Chávez, A., and C. Martínez. Value of different approaches for recovery of malnourished children in rural communities. Role of nutrition education in a very poor village. *Proc. 7th Internat. Congr. Nutr.*, Hamburg, 4: 246, 1966.
3. Chávez, A., and C. Martínez. Nutrition and development of children from poor rural areas. V. Nutrition and behavioral development. *Nutr. Rep. Internat.* 11: 477, 1975.
4. Chávez, A., C. Martínez, and H. Bourges. Nutrition and development in infants from poor rural areas. II. Nutritional level and physical activity. *Nutr. Rep. Internat.* 5: 139, 1972.
5. Chávez, A., C. Martínez, and H. Bourges. Role of lactation in the nutrition of low socioeconomic groups. *Ecology Food Nutr.* 4: 1, 1975.
6. Chávez, A., C. Martínez, Ch. M. Muñoz, P. Arroyo, and H. Bourges. Ecological factors in the nutrition and development of children from poor rural areas. *Proc. Western Hemis. Nutr. Congr.* III, Futura Pub. Co., Miami, p. 265, 1971.
7. Chávez, A., C. Martínez, R. Ramos-Galván, M. Coronado, H. Bourges, D. Díaz, S. Basta, M. Nieves, and O. Garcidueñas. Nutrition and development of infants from poor rural areas. IV. Differences by sex in weight gain during the first year of life according to their milk consumption. *Nutr. Rep. Internat.* 7: 603, 1973.
8. Chávez, A., C. Martínez, and T. Yaschine. The importance of nutrition and stimuli on child mental and social development. In *Symp. Swedish Nutr. Found.*, XII, Almqvist and Wiksell, Uppsala, 1974, p. 211.
9. Chávez, A., C. Martínez, and T. Yaschine. Nutrition, behavioral development and mother-child interaction in young rural children. *Fed. Proc.* 34: 1574, 1975.
10. Fromm, E., and M. MacCoby. Social character in a Mexican village. *F.C.E.* (Mexico), 1973.
11. Hernández, M., S. E. Pérez Gil, J. Aguirre, H. Madrigal, T. García, B. I. Escobar, G. Gutiérrez, Ch.M. Muñoz, C. Pérez Hidalgo, and A. Chávez. Las Practicas de Alimentación Infantil en el Medio Rural Mexicano. *Monografía*, L-24 (División de Nutrición, INN, México), 1975.

12. Martínez, C., and A. Chávez. La Nutrición de Lactantes de una Comunidad Indígena. Evaluación de un Programa para su Mejoramiento. *Monografía*, L-9 (Division de Nutrición, INN, México), 1966.
13. Martínez, C., and A. Chávez. Nutrition and development in infants of poor rural areas. I. Consumption of mother's milk by infants. *Nutr. Rep. Internat.* 4: 139, 1971.
14. Ramos-Galván, R., C. Mariscal, A. Viniegra, and O. B. Pérez. Desnutrición en el Niño. Impresiones Modernas, México, 1969.
15. Strum, S. New insight into baboon behavior: Life with the Pumphouse Gang. *Natl. Geogr. Mag.* 147, 673, 1975.

Henry Ricciuti **18**

Discussion

One of the reasons that I have been so attracted to research in this area is not just my interest in malnutrition and behavior as a problem in its own right, but because many of the issues really represent basic problems of concern to any developmental psychologist and perhaps also to any developmental psychobiologist. We are all concerned to reach a better understanding of early development and the forces that shape its course. Most of my colleagues in developmental psychology have tended to focus on the environmental influences that affect early behavioral development rather than the biological influences; however, research in the field of malnutrition and behavior forces us to examine much more carefully the way in which various biological and environmental influences interact in shaping development. It's important, therefore, to keep the broader perspective in mind when considering research in this area, particularly with regard to the planning of future research.

A tremendous amount of material was presented in the previous three chapters. There are many methodological questions, and questions of interpretation that might be raised about each chapter. Rather than going through a detailed set of questions of that sort, I want to focus on what I see as some common trends that are reflected in all three of the chapters in Part IV, trends in terms of the problems that are being approached and the way in which they are being approached, and trends that suggest important emphases on which we need to continue to focus as we move ahead in this field.

Let me try to identify some of the common ground. First of all, I think it is very clear that we are no longer asking simply whether malnutrition causes mental retardation in humans, or whether it causes impaired learning in animals. Rather, it seems to me, these studies reflect the fact that we are asking a broader question—

256

namely, what is the range of behavioral effects of malnutrition in both animals and humans? Can we better understand the nature of these behavioral consequences? Can we better understand the mechanisms through which these effects are produced? It seems to me that these represent very important basic issues that we need to continue to examine.

I was interested in Strobel's point, that he doesn't like the term "deficit," but prefers to think of the behavioral effects of malnutrition as representing a different way of approaching problems. This issue of more precise evaluation of behavioral consequences is a very important one indeed. Klein's work in Guatemala provides a good example of the much broader perspective which has been applied to examining behavioral outcome. The array of psychological tests that were used in his study is a very impressive battery, as is the range of behaviors included in Strobel's work. On the other hand, while emphasizing the need to examine a wide range of behavioral effects of malnutrition, there arises the problem that the more behavioral measures we use, the more likely we are to find some significant effects, along with many that are not significant. It is important, therefore, to look more consistently for replication of findings in the same research program on successive samples, as well as across studies with different populations.

Another concern is the matter of how the effects of malnutrition interact with experience, or with the environment of the child. What I see here is an important shift in emphasis in many studies—particularly in studies with humans. Rather than simply trying to partial out the effect of environmental variation, investigators are asking a more valuable question: namely, how do nutritional factors and social or environmental factors combine or interact in various ways to jointly shape the course of early behavioral development? Unfortunately, simple correlational analysis doesn't always permit us to answer that question meaningfully.

Thirdly, it is particularly reassuring to note that in the human studies we are making more use of experimental intervention, including nutritional supplementation. This is quite a contrast with most earlier studies, which were primarily retrospective in nature. Chávez's study and Klein's research both involved altering nutritional status by means of nutritional supplementation, and then looking for behavioral consequences of this nutritional alteration. The general impression that I have in reviewing the Guatemala work both before and after the introduction of the supplementation design is that this approach represents a powerful research strategy for trying to get at relationships between variations in nutritional status and behavioral outcomes. Some of the earlier studies, which were simply correlational, produced very little evidence of systematic relationships between mild-to-moderate malnutrition and mental development, independently of variations in the social environment. The results of the more recent analyses of the effects of supplementation seem quite encouraging. Although the relationships that are found are rather small, they seem to be consistent and to reflect behavioral changes that are associated with the experimental introduction of supplementation. How we interpret these outcomes is a matter for further discussion, but it seems to me that the use of the experimental intervention strategy here represents a real step forward.

I'd like to return now to the second point that I made, namely, the importance of looking at the interactions of nutritional variation and the social and environmental circumstances in which the child lives. It is helpful to think about this interaction as taking several forms. The first major form has to do with what we typically think of as a statistical interaction, in which the effect of one independent variable may be quite different for various levels of another independent variable. It is becoming increasingly clear, for example, that the developmental consequences of malnutrition are greater if malnutrition is combined with adverse social and environmental circumstances. I was very much interested in Barnes's reference to Blanton's work in Germany. Blanton observed that the children who were malnourished but came from better homes with brighter parents seemed less affected by nutritional deprivation than those who came from poorer homes. Most of you know about the Boston study of children with cystic fibrosis who were malnourished but came from very good homes, where the results showed no apparent nutritional effects on intellectual development.[2] There is similar evidence with respect to the issue of low birth weight, indicating that children with low birth weight who are raised under favorable circumstances seem to be at much less risk of suboptimal intellectual functioning than those living under much poorer circumstances.[1]

What is particularly interesting is that if we look at the data coming from the more recent studies of nutritional supplementation, we are finding that the effects of alterations in nutritional status produced by supplementation vary with the child's social environment. In the study by Klein and his colleagues in Guatemala, the initial findings strongly suggest that supplementation improved test performance only in the lower socioeconomic group. Although these were very poor villages and most psychologists tend to assume that such settings are quite homogeneous in terms of socioeconomic conditions, there was enough variation in socioeconomic circumstances, so that the overall effects of supplementation were found almost exclusively in the lower socioeconomic group. There is a parallel finding from the Guatemala study (not reported in this particular chapter) indicating that the effect of supplementation during pregnancy in reducing the incidence of low birth weight is also greatest in mothers from the lowest socioeconomic groups who were of short stature.

Interactions of this sort have also been observed in the animal studies. I was interested in Fraňková's report that the added stimulation provided by the "aunt" had a facilitative effect on various behaviors *primarily* in the malnourished group, rather than in the control group where the added enrichment had little or no effect. In general, then, it seems to me that this question of the interaction between variations in nutritional status, either occurring in nature or introduced experimentally, and the early environment of the child, is really a very crucial matter.

The second form of interaction between nutritional status and environment is one that I like to think of as a "functional interaction," which is perhaps best illustrated by the work reported by Chávez. His work is particularly interesting because of the close resemblance between the findings regarding the altered effective environment of the child produced by his improved nutritional status, and the findings reported by Fraňková and by Levitsky, Barnes, and Massaro. The general issue that we are focusing on here is that the altered nutritional status of the child may well alter his "effective" environment. This is an important principle that is worth reiterating, even though it is not new. There are two ways in which the child's effective environment can be influenced by his nutritional status. First, if you consider the inanimate as well as social environment the child confronts, the nutritional state of the child may well alter the way he approaches or transacts with that environment. This is the concept reflected in the earlier discussion of the "functional isolation" concept. Second, since so much of the child's early environment is social, we need to remember, as Chávez's study points out beautifully, that the way other people react to the child is very much determined by the child's own physical and behavioral characteristics.

The effect that the child has on the adult's behavior is of considerable concern to developmental scientists today. Psychologists have tended to look primarily at effects of parental behavior on children, but we are becoming increasingly concerned with the nature of the interaction between mother and child, an interaction which is obviously very crucial to development, that is also shaped by the characteristics of the child. Some of these characteristics may be biologically determined, as in the case of nutritional status, while others may be reflected in personality characteristics of the child. The common emphasis on this point both in nutritional studies and in more general studies of child development is a very important contemporary research theme.

The question of how to optimize the early social and learning environments of children is an issue of great concern to many developmental psychologists. Most early-intervention studies conducted by psychologists in this country do not focus very much on the question of nutritional intervention. However, with so many recent nutritional-supplementation studies now being concerned also with the question of added stimulation, I think that there is a great deal to be gained by these two groups working more closely together, sharing problems and sharing results.

One common issue that I would like to stress is the problem of defining the intervention, or defining the environmental manipulation. Levitsky rightly urged that we must learn how to define "stimulation" more precisely. I personally would rather not use the term stimulation because it suggests a rather passive organism being acted upon, rather than an active explorer of the environment. Generally speaking, we are talking about "enriched" environments which offer added opportunities for learning and development. In many of the early-intervention studies, one of the main problems is that of defining the "experimental treatment." If we are altering the child's environment through an enriched daycare program or an enriched cognitive stimulation program, it is crucial yet very difficult to define adequately the functionally significant dimensions of that intervention.

Chávez referred to the same problem in his study; while his main intervention was *nutritional,* he recognized that the auxiliary going to the home and bringing food every day represented a potentially significant added *social* stimulation. Also, the fact that the families are singled out as "special" may lead to additional supportive assistance to the parents. Similarly, in the Guatemala study, what about variations in attendance at the supplementation centers? Since mothers and children with high caloric supplementation attend the centers more frequently, is it possible that the frequent attendance is also having some positive social effects on behavior? This problem of defining the "treatment" plagues all of us who are interested in early intervention. If we can begin to define significant dimensions of the intervention more specifically and, perhaps more importantly, trace the mechanisms through which the intervention has its effects, we will then be finally on our way to a fuller understanding of these very basic, common issues. At the same time, we will be in a much stronger position to design more effective intervention programs.

References

1. Davie, R., N. Butler, and H. Goldstein. *From Birth to 7.* Longman, London, 1972.
2. Lloyd-Still, J. D., I. Hurwitz, P. H. Wolff, and H. Shwachman. Intellectual development after severe malnutrition in infancy. *Pediatrics* 54: 306, 1974.

Discussion: Problems Posed by Progress

It is quite apparent that a number of challenges have been presented in the early chapters of this book. These have not been completely resolved, although they have been thoughtfully addressed. We have, however, demonstrated the value of moving back and forth between animal and human experiments, in that each enriches the other.

This interrelationship is clearly shown in the longitudinal study in Guatemala. Klein and his co-workers originally designed their experiment around the concept that nutritional intervention had its greatest impact between the ages of 2 and 3 years. By the time the required methods were developed, results from animal experimentation had shown that pregnancy was the period of maximum vulnerability for nutrition intervention, so they modified their design and their intervention.

Similarly, data gathered by Fraňková, Levitsky, and others relate quite directly and obviously to that being gathered by Chávez. The two sources of data complement each other, illustrating again the relationship between animal and human research. Nevertheless, as pointed out by Dobbing and Levine, we must not overinterpret the animal data and take it too far out of context.

There are several groups of researchers working in the Western Hemisphere who are attempting to answer many of the questions raised by the animal studies discussed here.

Earlier in this volume Cravioto summarizes his project. It was strictly observational, starting at birth and extending to about 9 years of age. The implications concerning the family environment and parent-child relationships have been enormous, as have the effects on both animal and human studies. We have learned from Chávez concerning his study of nutritional intervention starting with the mothers midway through the first trimester of pregnancy and continuing with the children up to age 2 years; a non-supplemented control group provided a well-documented comparison. His observations about physical activity of the offspring have been most significant. Klein has described the INCAP nutritional supplementation effort, beginning as early in pregnancy as possible and continuing through the preschool years. That project presently is planned to continue for another year and one-half, until the youngest child is about 4 years of age and the oldest around 7. A project in Cali, Colombia, not reported here, will attempt to determine the impact of supplementation beginning at age 3, 4, or 5 years. In that study all of the children enrolled were undernourished as determined by biochemical, dietary, and physical growth characteristics. That project has two major components that draw from the animal data we have been discussing, namely, nutritional supplementation alone, or nutritional supplementation coupled with educational stimulation. Finally, there is a fairly complex design in Bogota, Colombia, where researchers have begun nutritional supplementation in the last half of pregnancy. Part of the group also will receive educational stimulation through the home, with a special effort to teach the mother better ways to use the limited available resources for the benefit of the child. Collectively, these studies will provide a massive amount of behavioral, nutritional, and health data which should provide an invaluable data base for important research and policy decisions in the years ahead.

In spite of all the research that has been discussed from these diverse but interrelated projects, we are still left with a number of questions that will require further consideration before appropriate wide-scale nutrition-intervention programs directed toward better child development can be undertaken in the developing world, and maybe even in our own country. I should like to review some of the major questions of special importance to policy makers and point out where these questions are currently being investigated in major projects throughout the world.

1. What is the relative importance of protein versus calories? This question is only partially academic. It is an important theoretical question which relates to metabolism, placental function, and the physiological basis of behavioral change. It also is a very important and powerful economic question: it is easier to produce high-carbohydrate foods than high-protein foods. If we

263

overestimate the importance of protein, we may be wasting relatively scarce resources. It would appear from studies of world malnutrition that the shortage is essentially one of food itself, although the nature of the necessary food may vary from country to country, location to location, and situation to situation. It is my personal opinion that protein alone has been overemphasized, but further data will be required to provide a definitive answer.

2. What stage of development is most affected by malnutrition? Pregnancy is currently considered to be the most vulnerable period. This conclusion is based on the relationship between nutritional status during gestation and birth weight, coupled with the problems commonly encountered by low-birth-weight babies. But is birth weight a functionally significant intervening variable in terms of long-term development of the child? This still requires an answer. What about the period of infancy and the preschool years? What about the school-age period?

3. If intervention during the school-age period does make a difference, what kind of intervention is most effective? Should emphasis be given to school breakfasts or to a school lunch program? From a nutritional standpoint, I question the benefit of a school lunch program unless there is widespread identifiable malnutrition. It has a humanitarian goal, but a good breakfast would be more beneficial. Either, however, may have a direct impact on hunger, and hunger may affect the receptivity of the child to learning experiences. That's a somewhat different issue from the one we have been discussing here of intellectual or behavioral development starting in early childhood.

In the school-age period, we also have such special problems as anemia or individual trace-mineral deficiencies. These have not been discussed here, but studies are gradually being focused on this area which will have to be taken into account in policy development.

The ease of providing food in a school situation is certainly an important reason in many people's minds for continuing such programs for needy individuals.

4. Is nutrition alone the most effective kind of intervention? What about environmental factors such as infection? Infection affects the utilization of nutrients by the child or the pregnant woman. There are data coming along on this from many studies. We will want to watch these closely.

5. What is the effect of nutritional intervention on social interac-

tion? The environmental stimulation question has been pursued so thoroughly elsewhere in this volume that I don't believe I need to discuss it further. Of course, the child's activity level will strongly influence family interactions and also will affect the school environment. It could be an important determinant as to whether the child manipulates his world so that it becomes a learning experience or whether he responds to a learning stimulus. I would also suggest that malnutrition relates to the long-term activity and productivity of the adult. We have only limited but very tantalizing information on this, but for policy reasons we need much more.

6. Finally, what are the long-term consequences of any of these interventions? We have been talking about results over a 3, 4, or 5 year period. What happens when the child enters school or leaves it, or becomes an adolescent or, later, a parent? Are the results temporary? Are they permanent? Are they overcome by an inappropriately structured school situation? There are studies which suggest that the differences in school readiness and receptivity apparent at the time a child enters school may relate to prior nutritional history, but that after a number of years in school these differences may be overcome as a result of the learning experience. Is this true? Several of these studies will give us an ideal opportunity to pursue this notion, and I think eventually the results will be of major importance. Furthermore, as we think about the long-term consequences of malnutrition and poor health, we must keep in mind their importance in terms of adult work capability and social competence. The latter clearly are related to the social and cultural environment in which the individual lives and the expectations of that culture toward the individual. On the other hand, productivity, adjustment, and social competence also may be molded by a myriad of environmental factors of which nutrition is one.

To me, one of the most important issues presented so far has been the recognition that behavior is more than intellectual performance and competence. I think if we pursue that one concept, we will have achieved a great deal. I do believe that the projects presented here will shed further light on the many questions that have been posed.

General Discussion

One of the major purposes of this book is to examine critically the research on malnutrition and behavior. Several issues have been raised in the previous chapters by Levine, Winick, Denenberg, and Smart. The following section was taken from a general discussion of these issues by the participants at the Cornell Conference on Malnutrition and Behavior. In addition, an opportunity was given to younger investigators to summarize their research findings. The material was stylistically edited in order to minimize repetition and to maximize clarity.

DAVID LEVITSKY: I should like to address myself briefly to the comments of Denenberg. I agree with him that some of the statistical analyses performed in the 1974 paper[10] were not totally appropriate. However, the best test of any scientific result is replication. We have repeated this experiment several times and, using the most conservative tests, have confirmed all the results reported in that paper. More importantly, others in different laboratories have also confirmed our findings.

Denenberg also touched on another important point which I believe needs expanding. We have restricted the malnutrition to the preweaning period because results from the brain studies showed this period to be most vulnerable to the effects of malnutrition. In the design of our earlier studies we almost always prolonged the period of malnutrition 3 or 4 weeks into the postweaning period, not with the idea that malnutrition during the postweaning period would have any effect on behavior, per se, but rather than the results would enhance the preweaning effect.

When we started to examine the functional-isolation hypothesis, it was then quite natural that we would examine the development of behavior during the period of lactation. Indeed, we found many indications that the environments of the malnourished animals were different. We never interpreted these findings as indicating less sensory stimulation but rather that there did exist an environmental difference early in life which could possibly explain, at least in part, the long-term behavioral effects of early malnutrition, independently of a brain-damaged model.

Furthermore, the more we investigate this problem, the more we realize the possibility that the period of development between weaning and pubescence may be of even greater importance as a major determinant of cognitive performance than the preweaning period in the animal model, certainly as it relates to nutrition.

SLÁVKA FRAŇKOVÁ: As Levitsky mentioned, most of the work in this area has concentrated on prenatal and preweaning malnutrition. It is during this period of life that nutrition produces its major effects on brain structure. We now have data confirming Levitsky's suspicion of the importance of the postweaning-prepubescent period in producing long-term effects of early malnutrition.[7] We have very good evidence that malnutrition during this later period of life also produces long-lasting behavioral changes in rats. These effects, therefore, cannot be attributed merely to disturbances in maternal-pup interactions or to the effects of decreased DNA content, since the malnutrition occurs after most of the physical brain development is complete.

I would like also to comment on the concept that malnutrition may act as a general kind of environmental stress. In experiments where we carefully examined the behavior of animals subjected to environmental stress and malnutrition, we could observe qualitative differences in their effects on behavior. This suggests to us that malnutrition, indeed, is not like any other physical stress, but produces its own distinctive responses.

DAVID RUSH: It is probably wise to remember that effects on cognitive function now appear much less likely than changes in other aspects of psychological functioning. Such changes, induced by nutritional deprivation and present after rehabilitation, are more than just noise only needing to be partialled out before sound conclusions about the consequences of human malnutrition can be drawn. These other behavioral sequelae of malnutrition may be as important to the functioning of the organism, and to understanding the effects of malnutrition in human populations, as the study of cognition.

SEYMOUR LEVINE: Historically, the problem to which the early researchers addressed themselves was the nature of malnutrition as a cause of mental retardation. This is the reason why a cognitive emphasis was imposed upon this field. No one has stated that the behavioral differences observed as a result of malnutrition were not interesting; they may indeed affect a whole variety of performance measures. The difficulty is in trying scientifically to assess the contribution of malnutrition in a context which surrounds malnutrition. Essentially, you almost can't talk about malnutrition without talking about a malnourished environment. There is not one procedure which exists in the literature for producing malnutrition that is not grossly confounded by other environmental variables. These variables in turn may produce many of the behavioral effects. The field, then, is in a real quandary as to how to isolate malnutrition from environment even given the criteria of Denenberg's stringent designs.

STEPHEN ZAMENHOF: Malnutrition is too often connected with the concept of mental retardation. To me, and probably to the society, a much more important effect is the reduction of potentially gifted individuals to normalcy as a result of malnutrition. Unfortunately, being normal is not considered a disease, but for the society this is probably a much greater loss than the occurrence of mentally retarded individuals. There is no study on this subject, but logically it is just as probable to reduce the IQ from 140 to 100 by malnutrition, as it is to reduce it from 100 to the level of mental retardation.

HENRY RICCIUTI: I should like to ask Denenberg: Do you see anything wrong with the logic of the approach that involves adding experience, either in the form of nonsocial stimulation or in the form of the aunt, as Fraňková did, and looking at the outcomes in terms of behavior, as a test of the functional isolation hypothesis? Assuming that the statistics are correct, and the design characteristics are right, this approach provides fairly persuasive data in support of the idea of functional isolation.

VICTOR DENENBERG: My concern with the functional-isolation hypothesis is with the word isolation. It is a terribly dangerous word. It has an adverse connotation of "at risk" to it. I will go along with the notion that malnourished animals are functionally different, but not necessarily isolated. If you observe them, there is a lot of interaction occurring, possibly because they are packed together by the mother. However, the conclusion that they are not exploring the environment is a judgment made by the observer. It is an hypothesis. It is one that I can challenge and which can only be settled by empirical evidence.

I would prefer to use a word like "different" rather than "isolation," since it is a more neutral term, without the connotation of "at risk." I do agree that a productive approach is to do what Franková, Levitsky, and we have done, that is, to look at the interactive behavior patterns which result from malnutrition.

OSCAR RESNICK: I would like to challenge a notion that has been touched upon by Dobbing, Levine, Levitsky, Smart, Denenberg, and others. This notion is that the brain is not "damaged" by malnutrition. We have examined various brain cells from animals malnourished from conception. At day 30 of life it is very easy to distinguish the control Purkinje cell from the malnourished Purkinje cell; the control basket cell from the malnourished basket cell; and the control granule cell from the malnourished granule cell. Differences can also be clearly seen in spine density and arboration of the pyramidal cells. There is approximately a 30 percent reduction in the spines. This is clear structural damage to the brain, damage to the "hardware," as a result of malnutrition.

SANDRA WIENER: The issue is not whether malnutrition produces changes in brain "hardware," such as DNA or brain amines. The point of dispute is whether these alterations in structure mean anything functionally. We have not been able to demonstrate overwhelming changes in behavior under the same conditions which produce these obvious changes in brain structure. Instead of demonstrating irreversible damage, I believe what we are seeing is an example of amazing resiliency and plasticity, particularly upon recovery. We are not surprised by the concurrent effects of malnutrition on behavior, but are amazed at the lack of difference upon rehabilitation.

MYRON WINICK: If one were to examine carefully the data of about 20 years ago relating any of the structural changes in the brain to severe early malnutrition, one would have to say it was amazing that malnutrition had really no, or very little, effect. However, as researchers improved their methods and thought a little bit more carefully, the data became clearer that indeed very great structural and chemical changes result from malnutrition, a position that no one here today would dispute. This is the story of science. I suggest that the same thing will happen as we sharpen up our methods of looking at the functional parameters of early malnutrition. I am not surprised that one research group is able to demonstrate many changes in behavior and others have more difficulty in demonstrating these changes. We are in the process of developing our tools. The process of developing our tools is not restricted to behavior tools, but our neurochemical tools as well.

STEPHEN ZAMENHOF: If we cannot find malnutrition-induced changes in brain or behavior at a later age when we can demonstrate it at birth, it may not be plasticity; it may be only our ignorance. We currently do not have the methods to demonstrate histological fine changes, such as differences in the relations between various layers in the cortex. The differences in environmental experience must alter brain structure even though gross analysis may not show it. It is not the plasticity of the brain that is questioned, it is our ability to demonstrate the lack of plasticity.

DAVID RUSH: I am not sure that I agree with the argument that structural changes must necessarily lead to functional differences, and that the reason we cannot consistently demonstrate functional change may be not only because our tools are not sufficiently sensitive, but because there are none. There are a number of examples in human biology where clear structural alterations do not necessarily result in functional differences. For example, for any given depression of fetal growth the effects of smoking in pregnancy upon perinatal mortality are much greater in the lower socioeconomic class than in the middle class, that is, the middle classes are protected from this particular functional consequence of severe structural alteration. In this instance, the functional consequences of structural differences may be greatly modified by other factors. Thus, it is possible that parallel factors may modify the functional consequence of structural changes induced by malnutrition.

VICTOR DENENBERG: Let me speak from my perspective as a non-nutritionist and a long-time researcher in the area of early experience research. We have known for 15 or so years that very minor periodic events such as handling a rat for a couple minutes a day for a few days, or shocking the rat for one day, or exposing the rat to cold on one day after birth is sufficient to give us clearly measurable changes at the behavioral and physiological level on a whole host of parameters. Since those kinds of events can clearly be picked up in open-field tests, in shuttle-box learning tests, and by avoidance-conditioning tests of one sort or another, we know that our behavioral assays are sufficient. That those assays do not pick up effects of early malnutrition, raises the question to me as to whether the rat is a very good model for studying malnutrition. I am willing to believe that malnutrition in humans really does have very enormous effects, but the rat may be the wrong species to use as an animal model.

DAVID LEVITSKY: There are several factors which have contributed to the skepticism concerning the functional significance of early malnutrition; the most prominent is the inability of several research groups to replicate the findings of others. We believe one of the most important factors in demonstrating long-term effects of early malnutrition is the housing condition of the animals. Most of those studies that clearly demonstrate long-term effects of early malnutrition, including those from our laboratory, report that they raise their animals individually and with a minimum of experimenter interactions. Those studies that have been unable to demonstrate reliably such an effect rear animals in group cages. We have previously shown that raising malnourished animals in a "stimulating" environment greatly ameliorates the behavioral effects of malnutrition. We now have evidence that raising animals in an environment consisting of only two animals to a cage is sufficient to override most of the effects of early malnutrition. Thus, strict environmental controls are very important.

A second and perplexing problem is the sloppy way we interpret behavior. We use words such as emotionality, curiosity, and learning very loosely and base the conclusions that these dimensions of behavior are altered on single tests. Part of this problem is not our own inadequacy. We are forced to use common behavioral terms in order to communicate with each other, particularly across disciplines. However, we are just looking for arguments when we interpret increased latency to retrieve young as an indication of a poorer mother, or lower asymptotic level of accuracy in a discrimination test as evidence of an intellectual deficit. It is not as important to argue over whether malnutrition causes an increase or decrease in locomotor behavior as it is to appreciate the fact that malnutrition produces a *difference* in behavior relative to the control group.

Finally, I believe we must maximize our creativity in devising new behavioral tests, new theoretical approaches, new methodologies to deal with the problem of behavioral measurement. Malnutrition produces very subtle alterations in behaviors. Those of us in the business of behavioral assessment have primarily worked with fairly large behavioral variables, such as brain lesions or drug effects. We have directed our attention at the analysis of behavioral responses because of a long tradition. But the question before us is one of cognition and, more accurately, development of adult cognition. We currently have no animal model of cognitive development, and few people outside of those working in this area are at all concerned with such a problem. It is our responsibility to develop one, so that we will be able to answer the critical questions concerning brain structural changes and mental retardation.

JAMES SMART: I agree wholeheartedly with Levitsky. In fact, I would say it is very clear that many of the effects of early undernutrition on behavior in the rat are lasting effects. They are every bit as consistent as the behavioral effects of early handling, for instance.

Levine and Denenberg have both suggested that it would be very nice if we could assess the effects of nutrition, per se, on the development of behavior. I agree with them. It would be very nice, but I am at the stage now of thinking that it is not truly possible to do so. There will always be concomitants, inevitable accompaniments, of the nutritional deprivation. I do not think that it is possible to truly separate the effects of nutrition from all other environmental effects. However, I do not think that this invalidates the animal model, because the situation is very similar in human beings.

JOHN DOBBING: There is one very important part from this discussion that has been missing, and that is the failure to take into account the severity of malnutrition. Most of the work in this area is concerned with malnourishing the animals during the period of rapid brain development in order to assess damage to brain hardware. In order to demonstrate these brain changes we must use a very severe level of malnutrition. A comparable degree of malnutrition does not exist in human populations, particularly in fetal life. You can produce it experimentally in animals, but it's unrealistic in terms of the human condition. The animals at this stage (at weaning) in our experiments are about half the weight of the controls. Perhaps we should turn our attention to examining the effects of less severe forms of malnutrition on animal behavior.

MYRON WINICK: I think that Dobbing has really put his finger on an extremely important point: Can prenatal malnutrition be sufficiently severe to cause the kinds of effects that people are concerned about? I would also like to ask whether you can measure the severity of fetal malnutrition by what goes into the mother's mouth. Perhaps the physiological disturbances produced in the mother by mild, moderate, or severe malnutrition may be at least as important to fetal development as the lack of maternally ingested nutrients.

General Discussion

STEPHEN RICHARDSON: I would like to remind you of the point that was made by Sir Dugald Baird, professor of obstetrics at Aberdeen. He emphasized that the conditions of childbearing are largely laid down during the early childhood and adolescence of the woman and that by the time they come to be pregnant the conditions are largely preset. We seem to have ignored the whole developmental course of the mother prior to pregnancy, and are leaving out an important set of variables. Furthermore, Baird said that one has to look at the whole reproductive cycle on an intergenerational basis. Single generations do not start de novo, whether we are dealing with animals or humans. We are dealing with a generational process, and I think again we have been mistaken in restricting ourselves to such a short period of observation and experimentation. Herbert Birch made the suggestion that if a mother has had good nutrition and good health up to the point of conception, she may be able to stand a severe degree of malnutrition during the period of pregnancy without adverse effects on her child. On the other hand, if she has been chronically underfed throughout her lifetime and has had poor health, the same degree of malnutrition could during pregnancy have severe consequences for the child.

HERMAN EPSTEIN: I should like to make two comments. The first has to do with the work that I have been doing for the last 3 years on brain development in man. A couple of years ago I published papers.[3, 4] showing that there is not just one spurt of rapid growth in the brain, but in fact a whole collection of them. I suggested that there were 4 in humans, roughly between ages 2 and 4, 6 and 8, 10 and 12, and 14 and 16 years. These spurts were about 6 percent increases in brain weight and about 2 percent increases in head circumference, which corresponds to 6 percent in brain. These spurts of growth correlated very well with similar spurts in mental development, and suggested a causal relationship between brain spurt and mental development.

This information fell on the scientific community with a very great thud, and essentially nobody believes it except me and my children. Nevertheless, there are new data from Japan, Russia, Finland, and other countries that tend to give additional support to the concept. All the new data show essentially the same thing with one exception. The brain growth spurt which I said is centered around age 11, is closer to age 12.

Through the courtesy of Gerhard Nellhaus, who is preparing a set of head-growth charts for pediatricians, I have located a large amount of data on the growth of head circumference. The increments in the growth of head circumference appear around age 3 or 4, age 7, 12, and one more around age 15.

The spurt in head circumference for girls is a bit different than for boys. Girls have a very small, if any, brain growth spurt after about age 13, but they have a very much larger spurt in head circumference around age 11 or 12 than boys. The developmental sequence of these spurts in head growth is almost identical among people from some 20 countries. This cannot be accidental.

My other comment has to do with my work in mice. We were interested to see whether mice have more than one growth spurt postnatally. One of the major problems in this area, however, is the enormous variability among mouse litters. We went to work to reduce the variability of litter-average properties of mice. This is a problem which is about twice as severe in mice as it is in rats. The variability in litter-average body weight at age 25 days for mice is typically around 40 percent, so that in order to make a definitive statement one needs many more than the 4-to-12 litters that Denenberg estimated to be needed for rats. You need perhaps twice as many.

We have developed a technique that we call equalized litters. At birth we equalize the body weights of litters both in terms of mean and the degree of variability. When we did this, we obtained a variation in litter-average body weight at age 25 days of 2-to-3 percent; litter-average brain weight variation is about 1 percent, down from (typically) about 12-to-15 percent. With this kind of reproducibility of litter-average properties we practically do not need statistics to show that we have effects of treatments.

Using the technique of equalized litters we were able to show that mice, indeed, have more than one brain growth spurt; they apparently have three: one occurs between the ages of 1 and 6 days, a second between 9 and 13 days, and a third between 17 and 23 days. Moreover, we have been able to demonstrate that a pulse of starvation (11 hrs/day for 5 consecutive days) has a considerable greater effect on brain growth inhibition when it occurs *during* one of these growth spurts than *between* the spurts.

ARTHUR RIOPELLE: While many of us are impressed by the effects of malnutrition, not everyone is. In a recent article in *Science* by Thomas Poleman[11] of Cornell, he says exaggeration of the extent of hunger in the developing world was clearly good politics for the U.S. Department of Agriculture, faced as it was at the time with increasingly bothersome surpluses. Sales or gifts of agricultural products to the lesser developed countries under Public Law 480 could postpone the day of more stringent controls or lower prices or both to American farmers. I raise this point because I think there are a number of subtle biases that may exist in our concepts of malnutrition, including the one that we all want to do some good, and the bias of scientific conservatism which limits attempts to adhere as stringently as possible to the rules of logic in order to deduce sound, unbiased conclusions. Those of us who are in this area of research must always be aware of these biases, for they may result in exaggerated estimates of nutritional requirements.

I should now like to turn your attention to another issue. This is the question raised by Winick of whether malnutrition has a deleterious effect on the development of offspring if it is induced during either gestation or lactation. The answer is that for the rodents there is very good evidence that, yes, it does make a difference. However, it appears that primates are considerably different from rodents.

A nonpregnant female monkey when fed a low-protein diet will lose body weight in proportion to the degree of protein restriction; she may undergo considerable weight loss. In contrast to the nonpregnant animal, the pregnant animal on the same low-protein diet, and eating no more per gram or per kilogram of body weight, will gain weight and produce an infant. I have suggested that this effect might be a sign of increased metabolic efficiency due to pregnancy. It may be one of several compensatory factors during pregnancy which allow the mother to produce a healthy baby under nutritionally adverse conditions.

Another compensatory factor during pregnancy is the length of gestation. A female monkey has a longer period of gestation if she is carrying a male baby than if she is carrying a female. Moreover, she has a longer gestation period if she is maintained on a low-protein diet than if she is fed a high-protein diet. We can see the effectiveness of these compensatory mechanisms on the birth weights of the infants. Male babies are significantly heavier than female, but the level of protein in the diet had no effect on the birth weight of these monkeys. We interpret these data to mean that the animals on the low-protein diets adjust the length of their gestation period in such a way as to produce a normal baby. This

275

interpretation is further supported by the observation that we could detect a small but not significant effect of protein intake on fetal mortality. Finally, in a very comprehensive set of behavioral tests on the infant during the first 40 days of life, we have been unable to detect any statistically significant effect of "protein malnutrition" during gestation on behavioral development, further evidence of the efficacy of these compensatory mechanisms during pregnancy in sparing the fetus. So what I am saying is, therefore, in contrast to the data from the rodents and from other laboratory animals, particularly those that give litters; primate data yield a quite different answer to the question of the effect of malnutrition during pregnancy on birth size, on growth, and on behavior of the offspring.

MARTHA NEURINGER: I have some data on rhesus monkeys that are different from Riopelle's, though not contradictory. I have been examining the effects of a combination of prenatal and postnatal malnutrition, in collaboration with Oscar Portman, Miles Novy, and Hideo Uno. We have looked at two different forms of prenatal malnutrition. One was produced by protein deficiency of the mother beginning either just before conception or on day 50 of pregnancy and continuing throughout gestation. The second form of malnutrition was produced by surgical restriction of the placental circulation; the bridging vessels between the primary and secondary disks of the placenta were ligated on day 90 of gestation. In both cases the infants were fed a protein-deficient diet after birth. These infants and control infants from well-fed mothers were all delivered by Caesarean section on day 155 or 160, a few days earlier than the average spontaneous delivery. Therefore, unlike Riopelle, we delivered the infants at a constant gestational age. We found that both the protein-deficient mothers and those with restricted placental circulation produced infants with reduced birth weights.

All infants were killed 5 weeks after birth for assessment of brain growth and biochemical development. Brain weights were reduced in both the protein-deficient and the placental-ligation groups. We found no differences in amount of DNA per brain. There were differences in the total amount, but not the concentration, of protein and of lipids specific to myelin.

At 2-to-5 weeks after birth, all infants were tested on a series of spatial reversal learning problems. Both protein-deficient and placental-ligation infants required significantly more trials than control infants to learn the problems. We do not know whether this result reflects a deficit in learning ability or a motivational or emotional change attributable to protein deprivation during testing. We are currently examining this question.

I have one brief comment about social behavior. We have been accumulating information on social behavior in protein-deficient monkeys. There is one critical difference between our tests and those of Zimmermann and Strobel. Instead of using social groups in which all animals are receiving the same diet, we have looked at mixed groups of control and deficient animals. In these mixed groups, rather than finding the kinds of increases in aggressive behavior that Zimmermann and Strobel found in malnourished monkeys, we have found decreases in aggressive behavior and large increases in submissive and fearful behavior that correspond to the deficient animals' lower positions in the social hierarchy. This has been the case even in deficient animals of the same body weight as controls, and despite normal levels of locomotor activity.

KENNETH SAMONDS: I would like to summarize very briefly the work that has been done in the laboratory of Mark Hegsted, Marjorie Elias, and myself dealing with malnutrition and behavioral development in infant Cebus monkeys. A parallel study of young squirrel monkeys is also being conducted in collaboration with Charles Boelkins and several members of the Boston University psychology department. We have looked at the effects of the type of malnutrition (that is, protein deficiency, or calorie restriction, or a combination of these two), the severity of the restriction, and the age of onset of the nutritional insult. In addition, the dietary treatments have been crossed in a factorial design with two environmental situations—partial isolation (which is our standard laboratory procedure of rearing animals in solitary cages within sight and sound of other monkeys), and an enriched rearing condition consisting of 3 hours of play with siblings each day and frequent human handling. We have collected longitudinal measures of nutritional status, including hematological, biochemical, and skeletal maturation, and a variety of behavioral measures, including the response of the animals to novel objects or environments, social interaction, discriminant learning, and measures of stereotypic behavior. Animals were tested while they were malnourished, in our early studies over a 20-week period, and also after 6 months of nutritional and social rehabilitation.

Because of the complexities of the independent variables and the large number of dependent variables in these experiments, I should refer you first to a summary of this work to be published by Elias and myself in the March 1977 issue of the *American Journal of Clinical Nutrition*. The results show clearly that rearing conditions are potent determinants of behavior; these findings are consistent with the literature. The effect of caloric restriction on behavior appeared to be direct and independent of rearing conditions, resulting in delays in consistent response to a novel object and inhibition of exploration. The effect of protein deficiency was strongly affected by rearing conditions, ranging from no functional deficit when rearing was relatively enriched to severe deficits when rearing was poor; protein-restricted isolates exhibited severely inhibited exploration and increased stereotypy. The finding of no deficit in protein-malnourished animals reared in an enriched environment rules out, in our minds, the hypothesis of a simple, causative relationship between malnutrition and functional deficits. The combined protein-calorie restriction produced deficits despite enriched rearing and more severe deficits when rearing was poor, suggesting influences from both types of restriction. All of these findings are from animals which were concurrently malnourished. The important question, as I see this problem is: Do the effects persist after rehabilitation? Our results indicate that the abnormal behaviors we found during an episode of malnutrition disappeared after nutritional and social rehabilitation, with one notable exception. The group receiving the combined protein- and calorie-restriction diet with isolated rearing continued their hesitancy to explore after rehabilitation. This is the only test, and the only group, which showed a residual effect of the imposed treatments. Whether this is a reproducible phenomenon, and whether it persists after even longer rehabilitation, needs further study.

SANDRA WIENER: I would like to report on some behavioral observations from our laboratory, on the maternal behavior of the malnourished mother. Anyone who has done this type of experiment knows that it is not a one-person task, and I would like to credit Kathleen Fitzpatrick and Robert Levin, as well as Seymour Levine, for help in running these experiments. On the basis of retrieval behavior the malnourished rat mother was reported to have a decrease in retrieval behavior of pups during a test period. Smart and Preece[13] reported that rat dams restricted to 50 percent of control-food intake showed decreased retrieval during the lights-off period. Fraňková[6] reported a similar decrease in retrieval behavior in rat mothers maintained on a low-protein diet. However, retrieval is only one aspect of maternal behavior and by its nature requires intervention by the experimenter. Simultaneously to Massaro, Levitsky, and Barnes,[10] we observed the maternal behavior of the undisturbed litter. We introduced an 8 percent casein diet to the mothers from day 14 of gestation through lactation. Litters were kept constant at 8 pups per litter, and nesting material was provided to the mother on day 18 of gestation. Half of the litters were tested an hour and one-half prior to light onset for retrieval behavior, and the other half were undisturbed.

We found a decrease in retrieval behavior of malnourished dams consistent with the previous reports. We also measured the nest-building behavior of these animals. The dams' nests were destroyed daily after the retrieval test. New nesting material was given, and the nests were rated one hour later. The malnourished mother did not rebuild her nest by 1 hour; however, 4 hours later all litters, malnourished and control, were found to have nests of similar quality.

When we observed maternal behavior during the dark phase of the light cycle, we found, as did Massaro et al., that malnourished mothers spent more time with their young than controls. This was also the case when observed during lights-on. All malnourished dams displayed this increase in time spent with young whether or not they were tested for retrieval behavior. Most of the increase in contact time was due to an increase in active and passive nursing. Malnourished dams, however, licked their litters less than control dams. We found a decrease in feeding and drinking behavior and an increase in rearing behavior in the malnourished mothers. Self-grooming was relatively unaffected by malnutrition.

In another experiment we compared the time malnourished and control mothers spent with the young when the young were subjected to a daily handling procedure or when they were left undisturbed. We found a significant interaction between handling and nutrition that indicated that malnourished dams of handled litters spent more time with their pups than malnourished dams of non-handled litters. This finding appears to be inconsistent with Levitsky's isolation hypothesis. The isolation hypothesis asserts that handling should overcome the effects of malnutrition. Instead, we have found that in malnourished litters, handling appears to further isolate the pup from its environment by further increasing the time the malnourished mother spends with her young.

JANINA GALLER: We have so far been considering malnutrition during a limited period early in life or during a single generation. I would like to discuss our work on the cumulative effects of long-term intergenerational malnutrition on behavior. We are continuing studies of the rat colony originated in England by R. J. C. Stewart.

The offspring of rats malnourished for 17 generations on a 7.5 percent protein diet are smaller in size than their well-fed controls. When the malnourished animals are reared from birth by well-nourished females, the pattern of weight gain is identical to that of well-nourished controls with no history of malnutrition, suggesting that there is no cumulative effect of multigenerational malnutrition on growth. Refed animals are also as active as the well-nourished pups, although the animals who continue to be malnourished are significantly less active than either the refed or control pups. Of importance is that the refed animals did not "catch-up" on more complex behavioral tasks. During the suckling period, we subjected the animals to a test of home orientation, during which we displaced the pups from the nest to other parts of the home cage and measured the latency to return to the nest. We found that pups fed a low-protein diet over many generations are less likely to return to the nest than are pups from the well-nourished stock. On this test, unlike growth and activity, the refed pups performed similarly to pups with intergenerational malnutrition.[8]

We have also been studying maternal behavior in these animals and have found results similar to those reported by Wiener. Low-protein mothers who have been low-protein fed over 17 generations spend more time with their litters than do well-fed mothers rearing well-fed pups. However, the well-nourished mothers do not behave normally when given pups with intergenerational histories of malnutrition: they spend less time nursing and in contact with these young than with normal young. An aberrant mother-pup relationship may well contribute to the behavioral deficits present among pups with intergenerational malnutrition which were reared by well-nourished females.[9]

DAVID A. BLIZARD: Smart raised the issue of the role of genetic background in influencing the effect of malnutrition on the organism. I want to develop the same point in more detail. In particular, I think there are strong reasons to suspect that the use of domesticated laboratory animals has led to an overestimate or miscalculation of the effects of malnutrition.

This belief is supported by the results of an experiment conducted by Falconer.[5] He selected mice for both high and low growth between 3 and 6 weeks of age under two different dietary conditions. These conditions consisted of high- and low-plane diets. The high-plane diet was the standard cubed diet in use in the laboratory (carbohydrate, 56.8 percent; protein, 18.5 percent; fat, 4.5 percent; water, 12.9 percent; ash, 7.3 percent), whereas the low-plane was produced by mixing the standard diet with 50 percent indigestible fiber. The design of the experiment is depicted in Table 20.1. The results indicated that the genetic selection was successful in both dietary situations; after 15 generations of bidirectional selection in each dietary situation, it was clear that selection for both high and low growth was successful on *both* high and low planes of nutrition.

The principal interest in this study for the field of malnutrition derives from the manner in which the growth characteristics of these strains were affected when Falconer transferred the two strains selected on the high-plane diet to the low-plane diet and vice versa. When mice selected for high growth on the high-plane diet were placed on the low-plane diet, their high-growth characteristics were not well maintained, and they tended to regress to the original population's mean growth rate. In contrast, animals selected for high growth on the low-plane diet retained their high-growth characteristics when transferred to the high-plane diet.

Table 20.1. Falconer's experiment*

Diet	Selected lines	Correlated response
High-plane diet	H+	Regressed toward population mean on transfer to low-plane diet.
	H−	Retained low growth on transfer to low-plane diet.
Low-plane diet	L+	Retained high growth on transer to high-plane diet.
	L−	Regressed toward population mean on transfer to high-plane diet.

*Mice were selected on a high- (H) or low- (L) plane diet for high (+) or low (−) growth from the 3rd to the 6th week of life. During selection, the correlated growth response of these lines to being placed on the other diet was studied; i.e., H+ and H− were placed on low-plane diets and vice versa.

281

The converse was true of animals selected for low growth: the strain selected for low growth on the low-plane diet did not retain this characteristic when transferred to the high-plane diet, but the strain selected for low growth on the high-plane diet retained their low-growth characteristics on the low-plane diet.

Falconer interpreted these results by suggesting that to produce a character that will be expressed stably in a wide variety of environments, the environment during selection should be unfavorable for the expression of the character. In this context, to achieve high growth that will later be expressed in a wide variety of environments, one should initially select animals in an environment that would normally result in low growth (in this case, the low-plane diet). Conversely, a high-plane diet would be the appropriate nutritional environment to select a genotype for low growth which would later express itself stably under various environmental conditions.

I believe these results and the generalization resulting from them have important implications for the study of malnutrition in laboratory rodents. Laboratory rodents have been consistently and deliberately selected (inter alia) for high growth and reproductive success on high-plane diets—just the conditions, according to Falconer's data, where it would be predicted that if they were switched to a low-plane diet, they would be expected not to retain their high-growth characteristics.

It should be noted that this is the typical situation of an undernutrition experiment. Rats, mice, and other laboratory animals consciously selected for high growth on high-quality diets are subjected to a poor-quality diet during important growth periods. The results of studies of malnutrition have been largely obtained, therefore, using animal subjects whose particular genotype predisposes them to showing a substantial effect of poor-quality diet. It is not simply the oft-quoted case of using domesticated laboratory rodents whose physiology and behavior may or may not be representative of the wild type, or even of the laboratory species. The situation is rather one of using animal preparations which the very process of domestication and mass production has channeled into classes of genotypes which would be specifically expected to show a pronounced effect of malnutrition. Thus, the typical experiment on malnutrition is biased in favor of finding a substantial effect of malnutrition because of the genotype of the animal used.

The implications of this situation are as follows. First, results obtained using such highly susceptible genotypes do have relevance for the particular genotypes studied. If, however, one is interested in the effect of malnutrition on population means and variances, then the information gained using a narrow class of particular genotypes is likely to be dangerously misleading and result in an overestimate of the penetrance or mean degree of severity of malnutrition on populations.

One estimate of the overall significance of this problem would be to compare the response of different genotypes to malnutrition. In this way, an assessment of the importance of genotype in malnutrition studies can be ascertained. C. T. Randt and I have completed one comparison of the behavioral consequences of protein restriction for the first 42 days of life in C57BL/6J and DBA/2J mice.[2] Following rehabilitation for at least 7 weeks on a standard laboratory diet, we found that previously malnourished C57BL/6J mice showed a significant depression of open-field activity and exploratory behavior and an increase in open-field defecation. These effects were not seen in similarly treated DBA/2J mice. In this extremely limited context, it does appear that genetic influences do limit the influence of malnutrition as far as its behavioral effects are concerned. Such interactions between genotype and malnutrition may explain some of the discrepancies in experimental findings referred to recently by Smart and Dobbing.[12] However, to account for many apparent discrepancies, it is probably only necessary to refer to differences in procedures used by different investigators.

Such genetic studies should be extended to an evaluation of genetic limitations on the effect of malnutrition on biochemical and physiological processes. For example: Are effects of nutritional restriction on cell number and cell size expressed to the same degree regardless of the genetic background upon which they are imposed?

The use of inbred strains to evaluate genetic limitations on the effect of malnutrition is one response to the problem. However, this may not be an adequate response: inbred lines, although differing genetically from each other, may have all lost crucially important alleles capable of influencing response to low-plane diets during domestication. In addition, they are generally considered particularly sensitive to environmental insults compared with heterozygous animals. A solution to this problem would be to compare the response to undernutrition of samples of animals drawn from stocks of different but controlled amounts of heterogeneity,[1] or, possibly, to experiment with wild animals.

JAMES SMART: I would like to make a comment concerning maternal behavior, which is, in the light of what we have learned, remarkably consistent. It seems to me that the undernourished young appear to receive more maternal contact. Wiener, Galler, Massaro, and Levitsky apparently all agree. At MacMaster University, Ontario, Patrick Croskerry and Grant Smith have a most interesting thermoregulatory theory of maternal behavior. Their idea is, as I understand it, that the mother's ventral surface temperature determines when the mother leaves the nest and perhaps also influences her return to the nest. They first formulated this hypothesis when their animal rooms overheated during a short and sharply demarcated heat wave. They noticed that the lactating mothers tended to leave their nests and their young under those conditions. This idea fits quite nicely the large-litter/small-litter results of Leo Grota and Robert Ader, who found that the small litters had more maternal contact than the large litters, the small litters generating less heat. The hypothesis may also fit the results we have seen here, that malnourished pups produce less heat than well-nourished pups. This may not be the whole story, but at least it is a parsimonious explanation, and I think it is worthy of thought in this particular context.

SLÁVKA FRAŇKOVÁ: I have several comments to make concerning the work of Massaro and the Cornell group. In previously published work it was reported that the effect of postnatal malnutrition on lactating dams was to increase the time spent nursing or at least in contact with the young. However, an increase in maternal exploratory behavior in the malnourished dams was also found. How can both of these behaviors increase at the same time?

THOMAS MASSARO: The confusion lies in the definition of exploratory behavior. We did not use the description "exploratory behavior." Instead, we described rearing behavior and locomotor activity. Many researchers believe rearing and/or locomotor balance represent exploratory behavior. We make no attempt to define exploratory behavior. We do know that postnatal malnutrition increases rearing behavior, but this can be accomplished within the nursing area. We also know that malnutrition has no effect on locomotor behavior as measured by our observational technique. Thus, the paradox exists only when one begins to de-

fine exploratory behavior. The behavioral changes we have observed are mutually compatible.

SLÁVKA FRAŇKOVÁ: I would also like to make two comments
concerning the relatively small size of your testing cage and sample size. We use an observation cage approximately twice the size
of yours. This allows sufficient room for the dam to escape from
her litter and engage in many other behaviors. It is possible that
the small size of your observation cage minimizes the possibility
of competing responses from occurring. The use of a small
number of animals for behavioral observation can be quite
hazardous, particularly when one is using genetic variability. If
Blizard is correct, then in studies of malnutrition we may be dealing indirectly with genetic selectability. In our studies of behavior
genetics it has become very clear that large numbers of subjects,
from 20-to-50 rats per group, are essential in order to make valid
conclusions about behavior.

SEYMOUR LEVINE: I would like to make several points. The first
concerns the problem of genetic control. Genetic control for most
people means an inbred and therefore a homogeneous strain of
animals. There is another way to control genetically and that is to
obtain a genetically heterogeneous sample of animals. We have
been using this technique for years. We use the offspring of a cross
between Long Evans and Sprague Dawley. As a possible "human
model," this genetically heterogeneous sample is a considerably
more valid model than the genetically homogeneous one. In most
behavioral research, however, the genetically homogeneous
model is used.

The second point concerns the term maternal behavior. Some
have described it as latency to retrieve young. Others have defined
it as time spent in the nursing area. In some situations one can
observe a deficit in both. Under other conditions these behaviors
can be separated. The fact of the matter is that we do not know
what aspect of maternal behavior has important consequences to
the development of the offspring.

The response of the young to the dam *and* the response of the
dam to the young may be a far more important dimension of
maternal behavior than any particular response measured in the
dam. My own feeling is that what we are dealing with is not a
simple set of responses, but a process in which young have a great
deal of control over the mother's behavior. The mother's response
to the young during this early period may have very long-range

285

consequences in the capacity of the organism to cope with aspects of the environment. This may be the point at which the whole process of coping begins to develop.

We are in fairly general agreement about some of the responses of maternal and infant behavior to malnutrition. Now we must ask ourselves the much more difficult and important question of what these alterations mean to the development of the organism.

DAVID RUSH: We need to be cautious when extrapolating research on the laboratory animal to the human. This is true not only for outcomes but also for independent variables. Are the stresses on free-living human beings comparable in kind and degree to insults we impose on the laboratory animal? The research in animals is extraordinarily valuable, but it may be remote from the human experience.

DAVID LEVITSKY: The question of the validity of the use of experimental animals as models for the study of human behavioral problems has been raised by Rush. The question is fundamental and very important. The question is raised not only by many researchers of humans but by pure animal behaviorists. Both groups are aware of the disastrous attempts to use models of learning theory derived from rat behavioral studies in the classroom. The ethologists are well aware of the limitations in extrapolating from even one species of subhuman to another, or even from the same species in different geographical locations. As a result the comparative psychologist now most frequently asks questions concerning the differences between the behaviors of species rather than similarities.

In the course of studying animal behavior in general, and malnutrition in specific, we have made many naive mistakes. One of these mistakes has been to attempt to extrapolate responses from one species to another. The particular behavioral response has evolved with the particular species to cope optimally with its own set of problems. What can be extrapolated is not a particular response, but a process. I totally agree with Levine, that we must stop trying to define the specific structures of behavior and attempt to understand its function.

All mammals have the common problem of having to learn about their environment in order to function as adults. The closer the animal is to the human, the more dependent is his behavior upon this learning process. The particular bits of environmental information needed by the rat are far different from those needed by man, but the process through which it extracts the information, processes it, stores it, and later retrieves it may be the same. Perhaps if we could understand these processes in a number of subhuman species, we would be better able to understand it in man. I cannot think of a more important problem than that of constructing animal models of human behavioral abnormalities. Research into the biochemical basis of psychosis and mental retardation, as well as cognitive consequences of malnutrition, cannot be satisfactorily researched in the human because of very clear ethical and scientific limitations.

Richard Barnes understood this well. Psychologists involved in both human and animal research must continue to work and interact if progress is ever going to be made.

References

1. Blizard, D. A. Situational determinants of open-field behavior in Mus Musculus. *Brit. J. Psychol.* 62: 245, 1971.
2. Blizard, D. A., and C. T. Randt. Genotype interaction with undernutrition and external environment in early life. *Nature* 251 (London): 705, 1974.
3. Epstein, H. Phrenoblysis: Special brain and mind growth periods. I. Human brain and skull development. *Devel. Psychobiol.* 7: 207, 1974.
4. Epstein, H. Phrenoblysis: Special brain and growth periods. II. Human mental development. *Devel. Psychobiol.* 7: 217, 1974.
5. Falconer, D. S. Selection of mice for growth on high and low planes of nutrition. *Genet. Res. Camb.* 1: 91, 1960.
6. Fraňková, S. Relationship between nutrition during lactation and maternal behavior of rats. *Activ. Nerv. Super.* (Praha) 13: 1, 1971.
7. Fraňková, S. Long-term behavioral effects of postweaning protein deficiency in rat. *Baroda J. Nutr.* (India) 2: 85, 1975.
8. Galler, J. Cage orientation in the rat: Rehabilitation Following Intergenerational Malnutrition. *Devel. Psychobiol.* In Press, 1978.
9. Galler, J., and M. Rosenthal. Maternal behavior in the rat following intergenerational malnutrition. *Infant Behavior and Development.* In Press, 1978.
10. Massaro, T. F., D. A. Levitsky, and R. H. Barnes. Protein malnutrition in the rat: Its effects on maternal behavior and pup development. *Devel. Psychobiol.* 7: 551, 1974.
11. Poleman, T. World Food: A Perspective. *Science* 188: 510, 1975.
12. Smart, J. L., and J. Dobbing. In *Ethology and Development*, S. A. Barnett, ed., Lippincott, Philadelphia, 1973, Chap. 2.
13. Smart, J. L., and J. Preece. Maternal behavior of undernourished mother rats. *Anim. Behav.* 21: 613, 1973.

David Coursin **21**

Concluding Remarks

In reviewing the contents of this volume, I am pleased that the major goal of bringing together the work of scientists from many disciplines has been achieved. Mutually concerned with the problems of malnutrition and behavior, the contributors have reviewed their projects, provided a forum for evaluation of data, and defined directions for future research.

Perhaps the most descriptive generalization that can be made of the information presented here is its "consistency." Indeed, there are a number of clearly consistent findings that have been repeatedly reaffirmed.

First, there is no doubt that malnutrition affects the central nervous system. Second, it appears that malnutrition and environment are biologically inseparable in their impacts. As a matter of fact, there is increasing recognition of the scope of the effects of environment on the development of the organism. Within this context, it should be noted that the term "environment" no longer is limited to simplistic criteria such as housing and educational stimulation, but includes a host of complex interrelationships—particularly of the family and mother-child interactions.

Third, reference to the effect of malnutrition on the brain is being considered in functional terms rather than in the structural terms that have previously been used. In general, there is little justification for using the terms "mental retardation" or "irreparable brain damage" in describing the condition of the malnourished child. These terms are political and public misnomers rather than scientific definitions. Actually, it is correct to consider the malnourished child as having impairment of brain function for age. Furthermore, it is increasingly evident that in most instances the condition is reversible, and that with appropriate and timely therapy catch-up and achievement of reasonable normalcy can be expected.

Finally, there is a significant concern for searching out mechanisms on comprehensive, integrative theory and constructs to conceptually encompass a broad range of information. Consideration should be given, also, to suggestions for further strengthening the capabilities for research in this field. First, a useful format for sharing information should be devised. While the meeting structure serves its purpose beautifully, the approach is limited in its capacity to develop solutions for the problems that have been posed. Interaction and productivity could be greatly augmented by small workshops of investigators that would include the participation of selected experts from specific disciplines who may have had no experience with nutritional problems, but whose personal expertise could provide a critical evaluation of current methodologies as well as recommendations for new approaches. A group so constituted could be charged with the responsibility for formulating research projects, structuring appropriate designs to be implemented, and identifying scientists most competent to undertake them. This is the kind of approach that is currently serving admirably as a means of developing well-engineered programs to provide solutions to difficult multidisciplinary problems.

A second suggestion to consider is the need for responsible concern on the part of the disciplines involved. Each discipline has a number of shortcomings that are understood by its members. In multidisciplinary studies, however, these limitations are compounded and may hamper the usefulness of a particular discipline in a collaborative effort. Hence, each discipline has a serious responsibility to assess its own abilities in order to maximize its realistic potential contribution in a multidisciplinary project.

On all of these points, the contributors to this volume have provided an important learning experience and a perspective on current information and future needs for pursuing the clinical, research, and bureaucratic aspects of malnutrition, learning, and behavior.

SUBJECT INDEX

AUTHOR INDEX

Malnutrition, Environment
and Behavior

Designed by Elizabeth Leah Anderson.
Composed by The Composing Room of Michigan, Inc.
in 10 point VIP Melior, with display in Helvetica.
Printed offset by Thomson-Shore, Inc.
on Warren's No. 66 Antique Offset text, 50 lb. basis.
Bound by John H. Dekker & Sons, Inc., in Holliston book cloth
and stamped in All Purpose foil.

Library of Congress Cataloging in Publication Data
(For library cataloging purposes only)

Main entry under title:
Malnutrition, environment, and behavior.

"Originated in the proceedings of the Cornell Conference on Malnutrition and Behavior held November, 1975."
Includes bibliographical references and index.
1. Malnutrition—Congresses. 2. Children—Growth—Congresses.
3. Developmental psychology—Congresses. I. Levitsky, David A. II. Cornell Conference on Malnutrition and Behavior, Cornell University, 1975.
RC623.M34   616.3'9   78-58016
ISBN 0-8014-1045-2